Nature's Detox Plan™

A Program for Physical and Emotional Detoxification

Designed by Nature
Researched by a Rocket Scientist

Roy Mankovitz, BS, JD, CNC

Montecito Wellness LLC
Santa Barbara

Notices

The information contained in this book is based upon the research and personal experience of the author. It is not intended as a substitute for consulting with your physician or other healthcare providers. If you choose to follow any of the ideas in this book, you might want to consider first consulting with your doctor about the appropriateness of these suggestions for your particular situation. Nature, not the author, is responsible for any positive (or adverse) effects or consequences resulting from the use of the suggestions or procedures discussed in this book.

Portions of the material presented in this book are the subject of US and foreign issued patents and pending patent applications. No license is granted to the purchaser or reader of this book or to any other individual or entity to commercially or otherwise exploit or offer to others any of these inventions, some of which are listed in Appendix A of this book. The following are trademarks of the author or publisher, or used under license: The Original Diet™, Nature's Detox Plan™, The Wellness Project™, The Wellness Diet™, Hypothesis for Health™, A Rocket Scientist's Blueprint for Health™, The Dirt Diet™, Officizer™, CellFrame™, Clayodine™, HealthBra™, ABC Food Test™, The Dirt Detox Protocol™, The Mercury-Yeast Spectrum Disorder™, and Whispers of Wisdom®.

Published by:

Montecito Wellness LLC
1482 East Valley Road, Suite 808
Santa Barbara, CA 93108

info@montecitowellness.com
www.montecitowellness.com

ISBN: 978-0-9801584-8-9

Dedication

To my mother Sarah for giving me life, to my wife Kathleen, my children Jill, Alan, Miriam, and Andrea, my grandchildren Alexa and Jordyn, and my sister Toby for their patience and support, and to my father Benjamin and my uncle Solomon, both of whom had their lives cut short as a result of medical errors.

Acknowledgements

In the field of medicine, I wish to acknowledge Dr. Orion Truss, Dr. John Trowbridge, Dr. Broda Barnes, Dr. William Jefferies, Dr. Laszlo Belenyessy, Dr. Hans Gruenn and his wife Annika, Dr. Deitrich Klinghardt, Dr. Michael Gershon, Dr. Guy Abraham, Dr. David Brownstein, Dr. Jorge Flechas, Dr. Paul Dantzig, Dr. Mildred Seelig, Dr. C. Norman Shealy, and Dr. Lawrence Wilson for their courage in pursuing alternative approaches to research and healing. In the field of dentistry, I wish to acknowledge Dr. Weston A. Price, Dr. George Meinig, Dr. Hal Huggins, Dr. David Villarreal, and Leo Cashman for their courage in pursuing alternative approaches to treatment. In the field of anthropology, I wish to acknowledge Vilhjalmur Stefansson, Jared Diamond, and Cindy Engel for their pioneering studies, which opened many windows into our past. In the field of cellular biology, I wish to acknowledge Dr. Leslie Wilson and Dr. George Ayoub of the University of California at Santa Barbara for their research skills and support. In the field of emotional detoxification, I would like to acknowledge Bert Hellinger, JoAnna Chartrand, and Dyrian Benz for their work in healing the psyche. Last but not least, I wish to acknowledge the support of John Posa, Esq., and Dr. Julie Staple, Esq.

Contents

Prologue

Close friends often refer to me as a disruptive innovator, meaning that I tend to create, invent, develop, or otherwise come up with ideas that upset the *status quo* in a variety of disciplines. I tend not to be satisfied with merely accepting on faith what others have determined to be the solution to a particular problem. I love research, and make it a habit to learn whatever I can in an area of interest, and then see if I can step back and approach the problem in a different way, often replacing the old with something new and hopefully improved. From a definition point of view, a disruptive innovation is one that improves or changes a product or service in ways that the market does not expect. A disruptive innovation ignores the currently popular paradigms and creates new ones.

Historically, I have repeated this disruptive process in a number of disciplines. When I began my career in the field of rocket science, the traditional approach to modeling the behavior of spacecraft was to use analog computers as the tool of choice. I chose to replace the analog computer by emulating its behavior on a digital computer, and then proceeding from there. Some of the results of this disruptive behavior are listed in Appendix A of this book under my various NASA publications.

My entry into the commercial world of electronics was based on a bold statement that I had made to the president of a company that made electromechanical switches called relays. I told him these switches were not sufficiently reliable for use in long space journeys and other critical applications because they contained moving parts that could eventually wear out from extended use. I told him that if I had the time, I could develop an equivalent switch that had no moving parts, and hence not wear out. He hired me to do just that, and the result was the formation of a new industry that produces solid state relays and circuit breakers to replace the old versions in critical applications. Some of my patents in this area are also listed in Appendix A.

When I entered the world of consumer electronics, it was with the intent of simplifying the VCR recording of TV shows by consumers. That project spawned a feature known as VCR Plus that was built into virtually every VCR to simplify the recording process by replacing the old one which was too complicated. Along the way, I assisted in developing the on-screen television guide, widely available from most cable companies, to replace the print guide provided in newspapers. Now, those electronic guides make it even easier to record programs using a digital recorder. A list of my patents in this area are also in Appendix A, along with those devoted to making radio listening an interactive experience, a feature yet to be deployed by the broadcast industry.

In the field of intellectual property law, I chose to implement a different model aimed at protecting and monetizing the patent rights of companies and individuals, spawning an entire industry devoted to doing just that.

Being a disruptive innovator has its rewarding moments, when something new replaces something old in a manner that yields an improvement that is appreciated by those who benefit from that improvement. Then, there is the other side of the coin – those who are being disrupted by the new – the disruptees. By way of example, how do you think the buggy-whip manufacturers felt toward Henry Ford? You get the idea – the disruptees can get downright upset about some new idea replacing their cherished businesses (or beliefs), even if the overall result is an eventual benefit to society.

Well, with that as background, it now brings me to the field of health and the art of medicine, areas that have held great interest for me over the last several decades. The first book I published on the subject is entitled *The Wellness Project – A Rocket Scientist's Blueprint for Health.* It includes a discussion of how I first became interested in health, how I became disenchanted with the information and counseling I was receiving from those trained in the subject, how I started over to re-research the area using the skills I had previously developed, and the startling, unexpected, and clearly disruptive conclusions that emerged from this twenty year project. Not surprisingly, readers are primarily divided into two groups. The first group has been extremely supportive of the novel hypotheses and conclusions I have drawn (backed by hundreds of references), which in many instances are in opposition to the firmly entrenched beliefs of those in the medical, dental and alternative heath fields. This group includes very open-minded and prominent MDs, dentists, and psychotherapists, as well as people from all walks of life who have been looking for unbiased answers in these fields, based on common sense and humility. The second group includes the unhappy disruptees, some of whom make their livelihood supporting the entrenched approaches to health, whether they are mainstream or alternative, and some of whom are consumers who do not want to challenge the *status quo*, since doing so may undermine their fundamental belief system as it applies to health and the medical establishment.

I am in the fortunate position that I do not have to make a living in the health or medical fields, allowing me a totally unbiased view. My motivation for writing books in this field is in the hope that I can help at least some readers with their health problems, and I get great joy when I find that such is the case. Profits made from the sale of my books go back into funding additional research in the fields of wellness and illness prevention.

Now, about this book, *Nature's Detox Plan – A Program for Physical and Emotional Detoxification.* It is excerpted from the detox and lifestyle sections of my previously published book, *The Wellness Project – A Rocket Scientist's Blueprint for Health [1].* That book goes into great detail describing my history and research as applied to an overall wellness plan, including diet, detoxification, and lifestyle programs designed to reverse illness and maintain health. Some readers indicated to me that it was too much information to assimilate, and that they were primarily only interested in the eating plans, or primarily only interested in the detox and lifestyle (healthy environment) plans. To accommodate them, I created this book for those interested in the detox and lifestyle plans, and created another book, *The Original Diet – The Omnivore's Solution* [2], which is derived from the diet sections of *The Wellness Project*, to accommodate readers whose interests lie in that area.

Section One - The Hypothesis for Health

Common sense is not so common - Voltaire

It does not take a rocket scientist to realize that something is very wrong with the health of our present population, and that the medical community has not been able to reverse what seems to be a relentless trend downward with respect to the prevention or cure of dozens of chronic illnesses. The goal of this book is to present a program which is designed to reverse that trend, but in a very unusual way. Over the last twenty years, I have voraciously read everything I could get my hands on that had to do with health, including most of the texts used in medical schools. I applied the skills I developed in the fields of rocket science, engineering, and even law, to try to arrive at an understanding of the problems in the health field that prevent a reversal of the trend toward illness. It became clear to me that the medical community is primarily devoted to the treatment of symptoms, not the prevention of illness. In a pragmatic sense, illness prevention is bad for business. My years of self-experimentation and research produced the program that is presented in this book, and I have been following it for several decades with great success. My reason for now publishing it is in the hope that likeminded others might also profit from trying all or parts of the program to evaluate its impact on their health.

More specifically, this book was written for those who are concerned about illness and are interested in a program (designed by Nature in this instance) to enable the body to restore health. It may also appeal to those who are intellectually curious about a health program written by someone with a background in rocket science. They may wish to learn about it in the event illness becomes a concern to them in the future. Then there are those readers who like to self-experiment (which include me). They may find the information in this book of interest from the perspective of illness prevention.

Most popular books on health are directed to a particular illness such as diabetes, arthritis, cancer, etc. One of the unusual aspects of *The Wellness Project* (upon which this book is based) is that it is not illness, diagnosis, or symptom specific - a result of my hypothesis for the causes of illness. This hypothesis was arrived at by observing patterns found in Nature and making some sense of them, and here is the result. Virtually all illnesses result from some failure of the body's defenses (which I will refer to as *the defense system*). This failure can arise as an inability to cope with a pathogen or toxin that entered the body, as in the case of an infectious disease or poisoning from ingesting a toxic substance. This failure can also arise as an inability to cope with some biological abnormality that arises within us, such as cancerous cells forming tumors, or foreign deposits in our arteries. Last, but not least, this defense system failure can arise as an inability to distinguish friend from foe, whereby the defense system mistakenly attacks what appear to be healthy parts of the body, resulting in autoimmune diseases such as MS, rheumatoid arthritis, lupus, and the like. I discuss the defense system and autoimmunity in more detail below.

The common denominator in all of these instances is some issue dealing with the body's defenses. Rather than viewing the problem as a defense system defect or disorder, I view it as an overburden of toxins in the body that either interferes with the defense system's ability to fully perform, or leads to a malfunction in its performance. I define a toxin, sometimes referred to as a poison, as any substance, natural or human-made, that is capable of activating the defense system and producing a deleterious effect on the body of a particular individual. The immune system is a part of the defense system and is traditionally thought of in terms of special cells in the blood and lymph fluid, such as T cells, which deal with infectious pathogens. In addition to the immune system, my definition of the defense system encompasses the bacteria in our intestines, the acid in our stomach, all of the detoxification properties of our liver and other organs, and undoubtedly, other portions of our body we have yet to identify that defend us against a host of pathogenic and toxic substances. A hallmark of an overburdened defense system is chronic inflammation.

A corollary to my hypothesis is that if the defense system can be relieved of this toxin overburden, it is then available to restore and maintain health, regardless of the illness. Some might take exception to the above statement when it comes to autoimmune diseases, where a traditional approach to treatment is to suppress the immune system to alleviate symptoms, on the basis that the immune system has become defective and is attacking healthy tissue. I have an alternate theory with respect to autoimmune conditions, based on my research in the field of detoxification. The theory is that the immune system is not defective and is simply doing its job of attacking cells that, while they might appear to be healthy, are not. I will spend some time defining the word *healthy* below, but suffice to say that what the medical community defines as healthy is only so to the extent cellular defects can, or cannot, be measured. Put another way, I believe that the cells that are attacked in an autoimmune condition are not healthy, but are in fact infiltrated by toxins and hence deemed "foreign" by the immune system. In the detoxification sections below, in support of my theory I will discuss examples of how some detoxification strategies have resulted in autoimmune illness remission.

In this book, Nature is used as a template to unburden the defense system from having to deal with (often on a daily basis) a lifetime of toxins. In its unburdened state, the defense system is then fully available to respond in a proper manner to existing illnesses, and to ward off future ones. Of course, the extent to which health can be restored in an individual is controlled by many factors, including any permanent damage that may have occurred in the past affecting the defense or other systems.

My analyses have also shown that it is the defense system, not drugs, chemotherapy, radiation, or a supplement that ultimately cures the person. While medical intervention may assist the defense system in coping with the problem, the actual restoration of health results from the defense system restoring equilibrium. We know this fact from persons who have a compromised defense system, as in the case of AIDS, where no amount of medical intervention appears to be able to stop the ravages of illness.

The term *Plan,* as used in this book, refers to a set of plans describing how to operate and maintain a complex chemical factory – the human body. The overall plan, set forth in my previously published book *The Wellness Project*, includes a diet plan to put the good stuff in our body, a detoxification program to get a lifetime of bad stuff out of our body, and suggested changes in lifestyle to enhance our health. In every instance, in keeping with the hypothesis, the goal is to minimize the intake of toxins, and to maximize the elimination of any toxins already in our body. This is a good place to point out that foods are a potential source of toxins, especially ones put there by nature to discourage their being eaten. This book will not go into detail regarding diet, and will concentrate on the detoxification and lifestyle sections of the plan. The information on diet can be found either in *The Wellness Project*, or in my other book *The Original Diet [2]*. The side box entitled Hypothesis for Health is a recap of what we have covered so far.

The Hypothesis for Health™

1) Illness results from a failure or malfunction of the body's defense system.

2) The body's defense system may fail or malfunction as a result of an overburden of toxins in the body (including those from food).

3) The body may be overburdened by toxins as a result of a misalignment between the body's evolutionary history and its present environment.

Chapter 1 – Background

The word "detox" will be used extensively in this book. The word itself has many meanings, such as spending time in a rehab center for drug and alcohol abuse. In this book, it has a much broader meaning, which is to either remove or render harmless foreign elements and compounds that have collected in our bodies over a lifetime. They range from incompatible foods, parasites (usually collected from restaurant meals), to mercury (from dental work, fish, and vaccinations), to a host of other chemicals (from drinking out of plastic bottles, sitting on furniture made with toxic fire retardants, and a host of other activities). We will even deal with drugs and alcohol, but not in the ways you would expect. The drugs include prescriptions widely dispensed to very young children (antibiotics), and the alcohol issues result from a fungal overgrowth (Candida), having nothing to do with drinking alcoholic beverages, but producing similar symptoms. These toxins tend to set a limit as to how high our pinnacle of health can reach, so it behooves us to deal with them now.

In the chapter that follows, I document what I call Faulty Human Trials – a list of Trial & Error experiments concocted by humans over the last 400 generations and foisted on virtually all of civilization. These experiments are ongoing today, and in my humble opinion, either singly or in combination, are the causes of virtually all chronic illnesses because of their potential to produce toxins in the body.

Regard this book as a blueprint for better health, where we allowed Nature to be in charge. The sincere intention of my hypothesis is illness prevention, and for those already ill, the reversal of the condition. The approach is really a "one-size-fits-all" set of ideas based on alignment with Nature. They are designed to benefit the body regardless of specific symptoms or illnesses, such as cancer or diabetes or Parkinson's or acne. They are periodically detoxifying the body to eliminate accumulated toxins, and shifting our lifestyle to one that is more closely aligned with our natural heritage, while still maintaining most of the comforts of today that we enjoy.

Chapter 2 - Fooling (With) Mother Nature

It's not nice to fool Mother Nature! -
1970s Margarine Commercial

I like the concept of "Mother Nature." Somehow, I find it comforting to think of our designer in feminine terms – soft, comforting, and nurturing. Of course, She does exhibit some behavior that seems out of character – earthquakes, hurricanes, drought, a tiger taking down an antelope and tearing it to pieces. My point is that there are some things we like about Nature and others we do not and would like to change or at least control. We have an inkling about how She works (our so-called Laws of Nature), but for the most part we are quite clueless.

I would like to keep my writing style in this book as gender-neutral as possible, trying to avoid terms like Paleo Man and Mother Nature, so here is a shot at it. I will sometimes refer to our Paleo Ancestor as "PA," and to Mother Nature as "MA," with the caveat that we owe our existence to the fact that PA paid a great deal of attention to MA!

As a techno-geek, I have had an inflated sense that I understand how things work. I get a great deal of satisfaction in inventing and making things that perform, but these are not living things. My research into health has really humbled me. I have read many of the same texts used in medical schools, and it has opened my eyes as to how truly little we know about the world of *living things*. I now know that there is no way in my lifetime that I will be able to understand the workings of nature in sufficient detail to reproduce a living thing from scratch, or even to modify the way my body works in ways that Nature did not intend, without the possibility of causing harm. So, my best bet is to try to find out what Nature did intend for me, and to stick to it as closely as possible. The real beauty of this approach is that I do not have to understand *why* we evolved to eat certain foods or follow a particular lifestyle, or even to understand how the body works – it is enough just to know the plan. This is an enormous relief and allows me to concentrate on preparing the blueprint for wellness, which is really Nature's blueprint, not mine. My task is to figure it out as best as possible and document it.

The reason I have spent the last few paragraphs dwelling on Nature is in preparation for a discussion of what I consider to be some major experiments directly affecting our health. These are in the form of Trial & Error experiments conducted by humans over the last 10,000 years (and still going on today) that undoubtedly had and continue to have a major negative impact on the health of a significant portion of the population by directly or indirectly raising the body's toxin burden. One can look at these experiments as attempts to fool or change Mother Nature in ways that are supposed to provide a benefit to our species that Nature has not provided. In my opinion, we may fool *with* Nature (that is, we have the *ability* to launch these experiments), but to think that in our lifetime, or even over a hundred generations, we can actually cause Nature to modify her plan for us, evolved over 2.5 million years, is somewhat unrealistic. To remind myself of my relationship with Nature, I periodically go to the beach and walk out into the ocean, positioning myself squarely in front of a large breaking wave – very humbling.

Ten Thousand Years of Human Experiments

Referring to Table 1, I have listed what I consider to be some of the major experiments conducted by humans over the last 400 or so generations, which have the potential of adversely affecting our health and are moving some of us down the road to illness. However, for many of the winners in our society, some of the items on this list would not be viewed as a problem at all, because they have little or no negative impact on their health. For the rest of us, these Trial & Error experiments have proved faulty because their intended outcome, while initially designed to improve our lives, is causing or contributing to illness in our body by increasing its toxic load. In many instances, we have yet to recognize that fact, or if we do recognize it, to take the necessary action to stop it. One reason for our lack of recognition is the long interval between the start of the trial and the manifestation of the error, so that we have lost track of the cause/effect relationship. As part of this problem, we have also lost the reference point or baseline that we started with, leaving us with meaningless comparisons to arbitrary reference points. Another reason is our lack of knowledge of how the body works, leaving us clueless as to how a cause could possibly result in a particular effect. As part of this problem, researchers have confused necessary causes with sufficient causes for various conditions, and confused correlation with causation, leading to incorrect conclusions capable of doing harm.

I have limited the list (which if it included all of the ecological insults to us and our environment, would have gone on for pages) to those items that are somewhat under our control as individuals and that can be either changed or at least dealt with personally through reasonable effort, and which affect large segments of society. In later sections of this book, I will discuss many in detail, touching on the motivation for the experiment, the impact it has had on humans, and at least one way to "opt out" of it. In a way, this is an attempt to return to Nature's evolutionary experiment, picking up where we left off before we meddled with the plan.

Table 1

Ten Thousand Years of Fooling With Mother Nature

A Partial List of Potentially Faulty Human Trials

Eating Incompatible Foods	Halogens in the Environment
Chlorinated Water	Toilet Paper
Fluoridation	The Germ Theory
Amalgam Fillings	Antiperspirants
Root Canals	Tight Clothing
Heavy Metals in the Environment	Plastic Food Containers

As I mentioned before, all of these are ongoing experiments, so one must assume that somebody considers them worthwhile. These "somebodies" are very powerful entities indeed, including virtually the entire Western and Eastern health and dental communities (including a substantial portion of the alternative health industry), as well as food, cosmetic and chemical industries (and governments and universities) worldwide. They certainly do not consider the items on my list as faulty, since in many cases they form the backbone of their businesses or are major contributors to their income. There really is no money in discrediting the items on this list. To the contrary, there is enormous money at stake to perpetuate these experiments. How can toilet paper be a faulty experiment in health? (See below for the answer.)

Chapter 3 - An Overview of the Project

Life in all its Fullness is Mother Nature Obeyed

– Weston A. Price

The discussion that follows could be thought of as a roadmap that can be followed by individuals to reach or remain at a pinnacle of health. While diet is certainly a necessary element in the health equation, it alone does not appear to be sufficient, which is why I have devoted so much time researching detoxification.

Each of us brings to the table a lifetime of following a different diet and lifestyle, and each of us has a different toxin profile that can drastically shape the outcome of our choices. Add to this our individual genetic and other variations and the picture gets more complicated. Does everyone have to follow this detoxification plan to remain healthy? The answer is no. I am convinced that there are folks out there that can eat anything, smoke, drink, get little sleep, never exercise, work in a toxic environment, and live a perfectly healthy symptom-free life into triple digit years. They have acquired, probably by random chance, the evolutionary makeup that fits our modern environment, at least for the moment. How do you know if you are one of the *winners* in our present day Western society? You have no aches or pains, lots of energy, a cheery disposition, no illnesses, radiant skin, no weight problems, take no medications, eat whatever you want, and can't understand why others don't share your good fortune. Are you one of them? I feel confident that I am not. The problem with this view of health is that we only get the answer in hindsight, and since there is no dress rehearsal for life, I for one don't like the odds. I do not mind being a risk-taker in business, but not with my health.

Throughout the book, I will be suggesting literature and websites as reference material for specific issues that I discuss. Many of these references also contain additional information, in many cases regarding detoxification in general, that conflicts with what is suggested in this book. On the one hand, for those of you interested in comparing and contrasting differing viewpoints, this should prove quite instructive. On the other hand, I hope you will find the reasoning put forward in these chapters sufficiently compelling to place *Nature's Detox Plan* at the top of your list.

On a last note, viewing the information in this book as a change of lifestyle, I urge the reader to consider his/her priorities in life. This, of course, becomes a very esoteric and philosophical exercise that begs the question of why are we here? What is Nature's plan, if any? Reproduction is a clear goal of any living species, but beyond that, I have no answers except as applied to myself, and even those have changed over time. My personal answer is to set happiness as a major goal, which then shifts the inquiry to finding what makes you happy. As it turns out, Weston Price's statement that "life in all its fullness is mother nature obeyed" has rung true for me – I get a great deal of pleasure and satisfaction knowing I am doing the best I can to understand and follow a personal plan evolved by Nature. One purpose of writing this book is to introduce what has given me so much pleasure in the hope that it may do so for others.

Section Two - Detoxification

We need a Bill of Rights against the poisoners of the human race.
– Supreme Court Justice William O. Douglas

The purpose of this section is to discuss programs for getting the bad stuff out of the body, and it is with a great deal of frustration that I finally have written it. While this section is filled with some important clues from MA, it is also filled with a litany of technical blunders that have subjected many of us to needless toxins that read like a bad science fiction movie. The result is that, in many instances, the toxic load on our bodies has far surpassed what nature has evolved us to handle, and hence even her clues are not always adequate for the job.

At first blush, it might seem puzzling that there is not a major effort by modern medicine to research and develop detoxification products and protocols. If, as studies have shown, everyone on the planet, including polar bears, is loaded with toxins, from an economic point of view (if altruism isn't enough motivation) there would seem to be an enormous market, and hence profit potential, in this area. However, as an experienced lawyer, I have some insights into how exploiting this commercial opportunity within the health industry would have some serious financial drawbacks. Let's say a pharmaceutical company asked one of my fellow lawyers for a legal opinion on getting into the market of developing products to remove mercury from the body. Assuming the lawyer was astute, he might advise the company as follows. Since the company might make or have made certain drugs and various consumer products containing mercury (such as common vaccines), it could be setting itself up for one of the largest class action lawsuits of all time, as well as providing the general public with strong evidence of the company's culpability. In the field of tort law known as products liability, under certain circumstances, the doctrine of "subsequent repair" can be brought into the picture. This doctrine states that if a manufacturer of an allegedly defective product subsequently performs "repairs" in connection with the defect, this can be admissible evidence that indeed the product was defective.

There is a lot of tension regarding this doctrine because of its chilling effect on a company making repairs or coming up with remedies, which are usually in the best interests of the public, so sometimes this evidence is excluded. Because of the political clout of the pharmaceutical companies, I would not be surprised if they were able to successfully lobby for a special law excluding them from liability under this doctrine, and in fact they have been somewhat successful in doing so for the production of vaccines. From my perspective, the bottom line is that we are not likely to see any meaningful research in the field of detoxification in the near future, unless it is privately funded, and one of the goals of writing this book is to get like-mined individuals interested in pursuing such a worthy cause.

By adopting at least portions of the diet plans in *The Wellness Project*, and putting the good stuff in our body, one can take a giant step to stop ingesting natural toxins at every meal, thus relieving a burden on those portions of the defense system used by the body to detoxify. However, even if we eat the perfect diet, the accumulated toxic load of a lifetime can prevent us from assimilating nutrients, and also block and disrupt critical processes throughout our body, causing a great deal of illness. Fortunately, eating the proper diet enhances the entire detoxification process. Put another way, eating the wrong foods not only repeatedly toxifies us, but also interferes with our ability to get rid of both natural and human-made toxins already stored in our body.

In general, both a compatible diet and detoxification are each necessary to achieve health, but neither is sufficient in itself. It takes both to reach the goal. A body loaded with toxins cannot achieve full benefit from *The Original Diet*, and such a person might find that supplements and even healthy foods act in a paradoxical fashion, either not achieving the desired result, or causing an opposing result.

What I will be concentrating on here is in understanding and finding ways to clear from the body a lifetime of toxins that one has accumulated from environmental sources and from the medical and dental communities. The term toxin as used in this section refers to any substance that causes illness, whether organic or inorganic, and whether originating from outside the body or from inside. I refer to detoxification (sometimes shortened to "detox") as a broad term covering the processes used to render toxins harmless. These processes can include removing the toxin from the body, destroying the toxin and removing the residue from the body, changing the structure of the toxin so it is no longer harmful, reducing the amount of toxin to a level no longer harmful, moving the toxin to an area of the body where it no longer causes harm, and binding or encapsulating the toxin in a manner that it is no longer harmful even if it remains in the body.

In this section, we are going to look at major categories of toxins, some of which have been with us since ancient times and others that are of an origin that is more recent. We will then look at various detox strategies, beginning with natural ones and moving on to artificial ones developed to cope with modern toxicity issues. Had we not lost our operating instructions from MA, we would have known that detoxification should be an almost daily ritual, as it is in the animal kingdom, to avoid toxin buildup. For those readers interested in the myriad ways in which animals self-heal and detoxify, I highly suggest the book *Wild Health* by Cindy Engel [3].

Because most of us have lacked information on the subject of toxin removal, we are now faced with a toxic burden that has accumulated over the years, and is distributed throughout our body. The result is that, in some cases, the processes of removal can be quite daunting. My plan is to visit the various categories of toxins we are likely to harbor, and discuss natural and synthetic methods for removing them. Following the discussion of physical detoxification protocols is a section on emotional detoxification. Therapeutic protocols are presented that have a record of accomplishment for clearing emotional toxicities, which in turn enhance physical detoxification.

First off, it is important for readers to understand some basics surrounding detoxification. Often, it can be a slow and somewhat frustrating process, which largely is a result of the accumulated toxic burden we are carrying. Reading the side box labeled Detox and The Die-off Reaction will give you a feel for some side effects that are most assuredly going to occur. Second, keep in mind that patience is not only a virtue, but is mandatory in detoxification. Many of the toxins we will be discussing involve metals with very long half-lives in the body, some in excess of 30 years (the time it takes for the body to remove one-half the burden if no intentional detoxification is used).

Detox and the Die-off Reaction

A sustained detoxification program dislodges the body's entrenched toxins at variable and unpredictable speeds. Toxins are not only being eliminated from the system but also being redistributed as well. This movement from one place to another has the potential to trigger a variety of discomforting symptoms—different in different people with different levels of toxic burden—known as a "die-off reaction," or as a Herxheimer "herx" reaction. In some detox programs, living toxins are being killed, and during the process, they can release potent toxins, causing great discomfort. Discomfort could be slight, moderate, or extremely intense. Symptoms can mimic the original symptoms caused by the toxins, or present as a completely new set of symptoms. The classical ones are headaches, rashes, and pain.

There are support groups to help people through the process, and a few health professionals and spas specialize in detoxification. One tricky issue is to distinguish symptoms that are a result of the detox itself from those caused by an allergic or other reaction to the detoxifying agent.

From my own personal experience, I have found that slower is better in any kind of detoxification process, and one should certainly be prepared to feel worse at times, on the way to feeling better. There is no way to know total level of toxicity and how quickly the body can excrete these toxins, so trying to push the cleansing can wind up making one feel ill.

Couple this difficulty of removal with the body's limited capacity for safe rates of toxin excretion, and the timeline for some of the detox protocols can be very long. One informal estimate based on the collective experience of several who have detoxed is to take the number of years over which toxins may have been accumulating in your body, and divide by ten – the result could be the detoxification time needed to reduce the levels to those that no longer produce symptoms. Yes, we can be talking years –

some lucky folks can achieve some success in months, but it is not possible to predict. Once the process is begun, many of the programs should continue for a lifetime to avoid a recurrence of buildup. Detoxification should become a normal part of one's life, because exposure to toxins surely is. As we go through this section, various detox supplements will be discussed, some natural, some not, and some require a prescription.

Now that I may have scared many of you, you might ask why do it at all? Well, it depends on your current state of health, and your future expectations. In my opinion, the ultimate level of health achievable by any person will be limited by their toxin load. Unfortunately, there are no completely reliable tests to determine the overall body burden of most toxins in the body, increasing the suspense. On the other side of the coin, people who have gone through detox programs have finally achieved relief from life-long symptoms that the conventional medical community has been unable to address.

How might you know if you have been exposed to any toxins (aside from food), and what are the symptoms? If you have ever been vaccinated (mercury, aluminum, viruses); have or have had in the past any amalgam fillings (mercury); had root canals or extractions (bacterial toxins); bathed, showered or drank city water (chlorine, fluorine); eaten bread (bromine); used a hot tub (chlorine, bromine); live with commercial carpeting (bromine, formaldehyde); eaten fish (mercury, PCBs); eaten at a restaurant (parasites); been alive when fuel contained lead (lead); taken antibiotics (Candida); played on a golf course or in a city park (pesticides); used a cell phone or lived under power lines (EMF); drank water from a plastic bottle (antimony, BPA); worked around products enclosed in plastics (bromine), worked in a building without natural circulation (mold); used artificial sweeteners (formaldehyde, chlorine); or taken prescription drugs (the drug itself), there is a good chance you are harboring some toxins. The list could have been much longer, but many toxins and their sources have not yet been defined. The symptom list could go on for pages, and is expanding daily. The problem here is establishing a cause-effect relationship when we know so little about how the toxins affect us. I will try to identify some of the major symptom clusters in the sections below. Note that Appendix B is a chart summarizing the detox protocols, some of which can become quite involved. Appendix C is a list of resources for obtaining the various supplements and other products used in detoxing.

The body removes wastes and toxins through several familiar pathways:

- the kidneys through urination
- the bowel through defecation
- the lungs through breathing
- the skin through sweating

In the case of acute poisoning, the mouth also becomes a pathway through regurgitation, and tears, nasal secretions, nails, and hair are also minor pathways, but we will concentrate on the big four listed above, as they play a major role for conditions of chronic toxicity.

Chapter 4 - Natural Toxin Excretion Pathways

Urination

Generating and passing urine through the kidneys is a major pathway for toxin excretion. In order for the system to work properly, sufficient liquids and a correct mineral balance are required. I discuss water quality in detail below. Water intake is easily under our control, and an amount that maintains a pale urine color is usually deemed sufficient. Unfortunately, some toxins can so mess with the body that one's urine is always pale, regardless of water intake. These toxins can also mess with our thirst sensors so that we no longer know when to drink. Yet other toxins can cause frequent and excessive urination by causing hormonal imbalances. In many cases, it may be necessary to endure some discomfort until detoxification provides relief. A general rule of thumb during detox is to drink one-half your body weight in ounces daily, which is useful as a starting point.

Excess water intake can be quite harmful, since it can cause dilution and excretion of essential minerals. Some fruits have a diuretic effect we have yet to understand, and that can be cleansing. Watermelon is an example of a beneficial diuretic fruit. Because it is not natural to drink when there is no thirst sensation, one must keep track of water consumed, and make a conscious effort to drink a sufficient amount. During detox, sufficient water is important to the process, and dehydration is common, due in part to mineral derangements. One approach is to drink a glass of water after each urination. Sipping commercial bottled water, especially RO water, from a plastic container as a detox strategy is self-defeating, because the toxins from the plastic may completely offset any gain from drinking the water, which means you will be continuously increasing your toxic load with every sip.

There is an old treatment that has been used somewhat successfully for generations where people intentionally drink (or even inject) their own urine to treat illnesses and allergies. Considering that urine is designed to carry waste products and toxins out of the body, I would caution against using these treatments in today's highly toxic environment, as it may well have the undesirable effect of reintroducing toxins into the body.

For some people, eating certain foods such as asparagus results in a very strong urine odor, not very desirable when it comes to avoiding predators. So, I regard this as a whisper of wisdom from MA to stop eating incompatible foods, discussed below in the food section. By the way, this may also be a sign of magnesium deficiency.

Lastly, it has been found that the pH of urine has an effect on the excretion of toxins by the kidneys, whereby an alkaline pH increases excretion of some heavy metals [4] and may have other benefits. As you will see, in several of my detox protocols urine alkalinity turns out to be an important element.

Water

Water is an essential part of detoxification, and the kind to drink is fresh high-mineral water as found in Nature, such as spring water and the water naturally found in fruit. There is very little information available regarding PA and water, so I will have to make some hopefully educated guesses. In the tropics during the rainy season, rainwater would have collected in virtually every depression, including tree trunks and rocks, as well as in flowing streams. This water would have absorbed a high concentration of dissolved solids, particularly when found in rock pools and mountain streams, and would thus have provided an important source of minerals to the diet, such as calcium and magnesium. It would also have contained organic acids such as fulvic and humic acids, and certain healthy bacteria, all discussed in detail in the next section. I avoid highly carbonated water, as it is rarely found in natural form. As far as water containers go, cupped hands, folded leaves (chimps use this), and hollowed out plant parts, such as a watermelon shell, might have been used. Considering the climate and need for a lot of physical activity while hunting/gathering, I would assume PA sweated quite a bit and needed frequent fluid replenishment. I view water as perhaps the major source of calcium and magnesium for PA.

I do not drink water chilled or iced, and preferably not any colder than spring water, and I do not ingest ice at any time. For the gut to work correctly, it needs to be close to body temperature, which is where enzymes and other reactions work best. Pouring cold water on this process is likely to disrupt digestion, leading to future health problems. Modern water containers should be made of uncolored glass or ceramic, not plastics or metals. Ideally, only limited amounts of water should be consumed during a meal because it can dilute stomach acid, among other things, which also disturbs digestion. Drinking hot liquids with a meal, such as soups (like bone broth) or non-caffeinated fruit teas, can actually help maintain gut temperature. As far as how much water to drink each day, I use urine color as a gauge, and try to maintain it a very pale yellow, almost colorless. Below is a discussion of water filters and containers.

Hard water vs. soft water

Many people do not like so-called hard water, which is what is delivered by most municipalities. It is high in calcium and magnesium, which cause a white film on surfaces, reduce the sudsing effect of soap and detergents, and leave a plaque-like "scale" on the inside of pipes and water heaters that can eventually reduce efficiency and block lines.

Consumer discontent spawned the water-softening industry, where the customer pays for a service that replaces the calcium and magnesium with a sodium or potassium salt. Potassium and sodium are needed electrolytes in the body that are plentiful in *The Original Diet*, but we also need the other two electrolytes, calcium and, more importantly, magnesium (see section on magnesium below). The resultant soft water is super-sudsing slimy stuff that rarely exists in nature. While my shower door might look better and my appliances work better, what about my body? My priority is to my health. While I can always clean and replace appliances, I only have one body, so the trade-off for me is a no-brainer, meaning no soft water. I regard softened water as Frankenwater and there are dozens of studies worldwide that show a strong inverse correlation between the hardness (mineral content) of water and cardiovascular disease, primarily due to a deficiency of magnesium in soft water [5] [6]. A website containing a wealth of research on the subject is www.mgwater.com [7]. I would not bathe in soft water, let alone drink it. By the way, I will be using various terms like Frankenfood to describe a food or other product that has been so messed with by human technology that, in my opinion, it is no longer something I want to put in or on my body.

Before we continue with the hard/soft water discussion, I want to clarify some terms. Hard water usually refers to water with a high content of calcium and/or magnesium, generally in the form of bicarbonates. Healthy hard water, as shown in the research, is one that contains substantial amounts of magnesium as well as calcium. As you will see later, my view of the ideal is to have a level of magnesium that is at least fifty percent of the level of calcium. These are the waters that contribute to low levels of cardiovascular disease.

Concerning water softeners, new models of dishwashers have the option for a built in water softener to which you add salt, and I have no problem with this limited use. I know of some unscrupulous soft water marketers who scare people into thinking that the minerals that clog copper pipes will also clog one's arteries and need to be removed, an absurd bit of twisted logic. Without access to the copper-pipe-clogging minerals calcium and magnesium, a person would have no bone strength and/or be dead. In my house, I go to great pains to add lots of additional minerals back into the filtered water. From a water analysis, I get close to 3 mg of calcium and 1.5 mg of magnesium per ounce of high-mineral water, making available to me about 250 mg of calcium and 125 mg of magnesium per day just from drinking water. My assumption is that the water that PA drank contained even more of these critical minerals, so mineral supplementation becomes important, and is dealt with further below. There are many laboratories available to test home water and I encourage such testing [8].

Water filters

In today's world of contaminated drinking water, various filtering techniques are in wide use to eliminate toxins, but many of them also remove important essential minerals, or otherwise add unhealthy compounds. I avoid distilled water (I don't think it exists in Nature), reverse osmosis (RO) treated water (similar to distilled), and soft water (rarely found in Nature). Virtually all of the drinking water available to us today does require filtering to eliminate toxins.

Many healthy indigenous groups have had access to spring water packed with minerals collected on the way down from mountain heights, and sterilized by ultraviolet light from the sun. I do not think it is a coincidence that some of the longest lived groups live in mountainous areas close to free-flowing streams. In modern times, the water that reaches your home usually starts its journey from a reservoir, then goes through one or more treatment plants that add toxins such as chlorine and fluorine, then perhaps travels through an aqueduct before going underground through a pipe system. The pipes may be made of iron, plastic, copper, or ceramic, and the water picks up some of the particles of these materials. Alternatively, you may be using well water, which picks up all of the groundwater toxins that have percolated into it from human-made sources.

In order to protect consumers against bacterial buildup, since 1908, municipalities have been treating with chlorine the water they sell to consumers. Unfortunately, this element is toxic not just to bacteria but to humans as well. When chlorine reacts with organic substances, it forms compounds called chloramines, which are known carcinogens. Chlorine itself is a neurotoxin and interferes with certain hormonal processes, as discussed further below. Municipal water may also include variable trace levels of nasty substances such as runoff residuals of fertilizers, pesticides, herbicides, and fungicides, heavy metals, cysts, viruses, fungi, bacteria, industrial wastes, rocket fuel, and prescription drugs such as antibiotics and hormones.

Drinking, showering or bathing in this stuff is a good way to add toxins to the body. In a shower the hot water opens pores and we can inhale and absorb large amounts of the bad stuff (spas, hot, tubs, and pools add to the toxin problem with their use of chlorine, bromine, and algaecides; this is dealt with separately in the halogen portion of the detox section). Therefore, water filtering is a necessary part of *Nature's Detox Plan*, with the goal of matching the healthy characteristics of fresh mountain stream water as closely as possible.

One option is the reverse osmosis system (RO) system, commonly used in under-the-counter kitchen filters. The problem with this method is that it removes not just the bad impurities but a lot of the good stuff as well, namely minerals. Plumbers installing RO (and distillation) filters take care to be sure that the water from the filter does not run through a copper pipe to the drinking spout. The instructions for such systems, in fact, caution not to use copper (or any metal) for this purpose. That's because RO (and distilled) water will suck the copper right out of the pipe.

For those using an RO or distillation system, there are a number of re-mineralizer systems on the market that claim to add back some of the missing minerals, primarily calcium and magnesium, and they may be worth an investigation. Another approach is to take a mineral supplement along with RO or distilled water. It seems to me that an important part of the mineral content of mountain spring water comes from the rocks over and through which the water flows as it travels down to the ocean. A very common type of such rock is a form of limestone known as dolomite. It has a high concentration of calcium and magnesium carbonate in approximately a 1.7 to 1 ratio. Carbonate forms of minerals have been dismissed by the mineral supplement industry on the basis that they have a low percentage of assimilation in the human gut. If that was in fact true, all mineral waters would seem to be useless, and they are not. Calcium and magnesium in natural mineral water appear in the form of soluble bicarbonates, which are produced when the carbonate forms of the minerals, such as in dolomite, are combined with carbon dioxide in the water.

I would rather listen to MA than the supplement industry, and I use a dolomite supplement to replicate closely the mineral content of spring water. A few years ago, dolomite supplements had a bad name because some brands contained high levels of lead. I have found a source of dolomite from a supplier who indicates they derive their dolomite from deeply buried ancient mineral deposits free of toxic metals. They test their product for lead, with a limit of ten parts per billion, a very low level [9]. While there is no safe level for lead, magnesium acts to displace and replace it in the body, so the high levels of magnesium in dolomite mitigate against even these small amounts of lead as being troublesome. One dolomite tablet with each glass of water (not with meals because it can neutralize stomach acid), up to four tablets per day (a total of 630 mg of calcium and 360 mg of magnesium), would seem to restore a good part of the natural calcium and magnesium missing from RO or distilled water. I will be discussing dolomite further in the mineral section below, but I want to emphasize its importance as a completely natural compound, undoubtedly loaded with essential trace minerals. A fascinating book discussing the health benefits of dolomite was written decades ago by Jerome Rodale, a pioneer in the health field [10].

Although I am not a fan of plastic pipes, in the case of RO or distilled water systems they are definitely required. Copper toxicity is a much-overlooked contributor to health problems including rheumatoid and osteoarthritis, bone fractures, decreased libido, panic attacks, hair loss, fatigue, and childhood hyperactivity and learning disorders. These types of filtered water should not pass through any kind of metal, including metal water bottles or cooking utensils, as the water may absorb components of the metal itself. An issue I have with many RO and distiller systems is that the drinking faucet may be made of copper or brass, so the water sitting in contact with the faucet may well be leaching metals from the faucet into the water. Copper is an important mineral for health but only in very small amounts, beyond which it is toxic [11].

Unfortunately, RO and distilled water may also absorb toxins from the plastic pipes. Why is this so? As many of you recall from science class, water is the universal solvent, and acts to dissolve solids up to the point where it is fully saturated. Well, distilled and RO water contain virtually no dissolved solids, so they act very aggressively to dissolve whatever it is they are in contact with. Opposed to this is water with a high desirable mineral content, which is close to or at saturation, and hence has very little affinity for dissolving unwanted substances, like copper and plastic from pipes and containers. This is not rocket science. Which brings up stainless steel.

Most water distillation filters use a stainless steel tank (hopefully food grade) to heat and hold the water. Stainless steel is used everywhere in the food industry, from raw ingredient containers to cooking utensils to eating utensils, as well as in medical and dental instruments. Stainless steel is the name given to iron based alloys containing at least 10% chromium. I am not a metallurgist, but I took my share of metallurgy courses in college, and it is well known that all iron alloys exposed to water and oxygen will corrode, and a popular industry spec for stainless steel allows for 0.1 mm of surface corrosion per year. So-called food-grade stainless alloys include Type 304, which contains chromium, nickel, carbon, and manganese, and is known as 18/8 stainless. Type 316 has higher corrosion resistance, and further includes molybdenum. Stainless steel is also used in water heaters and water filters. Since it is virtually impossible to avoid stainless steel, my point is to raise the possibility that small amounts of iron, chromium, nickel and molybdenum may be leaching into the food and water chain, increasing the importance of having a filter that removes metals. This corrosion factor is another reason I do not use stainless steel (or any other metal) for water containers.

Here are my filter suggestions. Starting with the simplest, for drinking water I have used under-counter (and counter-top) filters made by Doulton, a British company, and sold by many distributors [12]. The main filter uses a ceramic cartridge impregnated with silver. Many other cartridges are available for specific filter requirements, such as eliminating fluoride, and the model HIP-320 is a good choice. In a way, using ceramic mimics MA's natural rock filtration system. By the way, the bibliography section and Appendix C at the end of this book contains many website references to potential sources of information and/or products.

For a shower filter, I have used the Shower Soft Filter by Hydro-Flow Filtration Systems [13], and it is easily installed in most showers just behind the showerhead. It uses KDF, a filter medium that works well in cold or hot water to remove chlorine and many organic toxins, so your shower (and you) will no longer have a chlorine odor. For those who like to take baths, the tub can be filled with water from the shower.

One of the most intriguing water filters on the market is called the Wellness Filter, a Japanese product line ranging from showerheads to whole-house systems that is designed to replicate mountain stream water [14]. The filters not only remove most of the bad stuff (fluoride is an exception), many models re-insert into the water desirable minerals mined from various volcanic mountain locations in Japan which have been studied for millennia for their healing properties. They mine the rock from those locations, pulverized it, and layer it into their filters, which also include carbon, KDF, and magnetics. Apparently, Japanese hospitals and some of their Olympic teams are using these filters, and high-end American restaurants have started to install them as well. I have a whole-house version of the filter that works well. It is programmed to backwash weekly, and no media (filter element) replacement is required for many years.

For communities that have fluoridated water, the filter problem is substantially more complicated. Eliminating fluoride requires either RO, or distillation, or a special media filter, so for those unlucky enough to be in a community that fluoridates its water, one of these filters would be useful wherever there is a drinking water spout. The media filter uses aluminum oxide, so there should be a KDF and carbon filter following it to remove any aluminum oxide that may leach into the water. The Doulton filter does the job with the right selection of filter elements. Users of the whole house Wellness filter, which does not remove fluoride, may need to include a Doulton unit at drinking stations. I do not know of any whole house system for removing fluoride, leaving one vulnerable to shower inhalation and absorption of this potentially toxic mineral. Alternatives are to petition local government to get the fluoride out of the water (it is a nasty toxin), or to move (I moved). I cover the fluoride problem in more depth below, where I also discuss water filters for hot tubs, spas, and swimming pools.

Water Bottles

The plastic water bottle is everywhere, and it is difficult to pick a starting point to discuss its toxicity because the playing field is rapidly expanding. Let's begin with the most popular plastic, polyethylene terephthalate (PET), shown as a #1 inside a triangle on the bottle bottom, and used by virtually all brands of bottled water. A somewhat recent study showed elevated levels of the metal antimony leaching from these bottles into the water [15]. Antimony is nasty stuff, and while the amounts measured were below the supposedly acceptable level, they were hundreds of times higher than levels normally found in drinking water, not surprising since antimony trioxide is used in the production of PET. There is almost no information on the hazards of oral ingestion of antimony, but it is a cumulative metal with a long half-life, and it is rated as carcinogenic. It also appears in breast milk, crosses the placenta, and may be a cause of miscarriages. Compound this with the fact that much of the bottled water is made using the RO process, so it is in a state where it can aggressively absorb bad stuff, like antimony. Over thirty years ago, it was reported that plants watered with water stored in PET bottles did not grow as well as those watered without using plastic [16], which raises all sorts of issues as to the impact on plant foods of plastic used in irrigation systems.

Moving on to polycarbonate bottles, these are the hard plastic ones that sometimes come in colors, or have a bluish cast in a semitransparent style, with a #7 on the bottom in a triangle. They leach bisphenol-A (BPA) into the water, and this chemical, which is also found in soup and soda can liners, is an estrogen mimic that can cause hormone havoc. It had been found in baby bottles, pacifiers and other toys, and because it can be particularly devastating to children, its use has been banned in many of these products [17]. Washing these bottles with a detergent can worsen the situation. I have seen people at the market line up with their re-usable # 7 water containers and put money into a machine that generates RO water from tap water. Here again, putting mineral-free RO water into plastic is not a great idea, and I wonder if there is any real health benefit for their efforts. So far, plastic containers labeled #2, #4 or #5 have escaped the toxic tide, but my guess would be it is only a matter of time before they too meet the fate of #1 and #7. This is not rocket science. All plastic containers are toxic.

Many health-minded people are switching to metal bottles, and stainless steel is becoming the vogue. I already covered the issues I have with stainless, and I would not drink from them or cook in metal. Other fashion bottles claim to have inert liners of one sort or another, such as epoxy. Most common epoxy resins are produced from a reaction between epichlorohydrin and bisphenol-A. We dealt with bisphenol-A above, and epichlorohydrin is a known reproductive toxin. Many epoxies are FDA approved for contact with foods, and they may be somewhat inert until scratched or otherwise abraded. Those who insist upon metal might want to consider drinking out of a sterling silver goblet (see side box below).

A Non-Toxic Plastic Water Bottle?

Many folks know of the potential toxicity of plastic water bottles, but are not willing to lug around a heavy glass one. I will be commenting further about the unique properties of silver, and certainly one could safely drink out of a silver cup. I came up with the idea of combining silver and a plastic such as polycarbonate with two objectives in mind. First is to use the silver to bind with the toxic components in the plastic to prevent them from being leached into the water. Second is to provide a source of silver ions on the inside and outside surface of the container to disinfect the water in the container, and to disinfect the hands of the user on the outside of the container, in an effort to avoid the spread of nasty bacterial infections such as MRSA (methicillin resistant staphylococcus aureus). I have filed a patent application covering the concept in the hope of attracting a company to commercialize it.

So what's left to drink out of? How about good old glass? Yes, it can break on impact, and it's a lot heavier than plastic but it's the best and safest choice, along with uncolored ceramic. Some flat mineral water products are sold in glass bottles, such as Evian, and they can be reused. Alternatively, glass bottles of all shapes and sizes can be purchased online from a variety of sources [18]. I particularly like swing-top locking flask designs. Cloth water bottle holders with straps are available to minimize the chances of breakage, and can also be used to make a fashion statement!

Defecation

Generating and passing fecal matter through the colon is another major pathway for toxin excretion. In order for this system to work properly, you need the colon to work as designed, removing water and some minerals from the fecal mass, and consolidating it into stool. We do not fully understand how this works, but it definitely requires the cooperation of the large biomass of bacteria and fungi and possibly some other parasites in the colon to make it happen. In fact, the bulk of the stool is made up of gut bacteria. The muscle system controlling the gut must also be operating correctly to generate the peristaltic action necessary to move the digested food along in the gut. Some toxins can seriously mess with normal defecation. For this reason, my belief is that in the future we will discover that illnesses with names such as irritable bowel syndrome (IBS), irritable bowel disease (IBD), and Crohn's disease are all various manifestations of toxin disturbances of the gut.

For those readers who are squeamish, I am about to launch into a somewhat graphic description of bowel movements (BMs), and I hope you will not shy away from it. As in the case of any chemical factory like the human body, it is very important to analyze not only what you put into the body, but also what comes out of it. Paying attention to the condition of one's bowel is a simple way of detecting intestinal problems at an early stage, yet even mentioning such a subject is shunned as culturally and socially unacceptable. The goal of this analysis is to try to determine what comprises the perfect bowel movement, in terms of frequency, consistency, odor, and color. Sort of like a Wellness BM! If we can do that, then for those who have a disturbed gut, we can use *stool as a tool* to measure our detoxification progress.

It is rather amazing how little research has been done in the area of defecation, considering its importance as a diagnostic tool. There is a funny analogy here. Much like asking ten nutritionists what to eat and getting ten different answers, if you ask a group of gastroenterologists to describe a healthy bowel movement, you are also likely to get little agreement. Just the simple question of how often one should have a movement elicits widely varying answers, with the so-called normal range being from once a week to several times a day. There is no doubt that what you eat, as well as your toxin load, can have a major effect on your bowel movement frequency. We don't know exactly how many bowel movements PA experienced on *The Original Diet*, and most modern indigenous groups do not follow that diet, but we can take a look at the animal community for some clues. Chimps are known to have multiple movements each day, but their diet is loaded with fibrous foods we could not possibly digest, and they spend most of their time eating.

When on a natural diet, cats, which are obligate carnivores, have one movement per meal, and dogs, which are mostly carnivores, when on a natural diet also have one movement per meal. From my experience, one BM for every meal is ideal, with a minimum of once per day. I would view more than once per meal or less than one per day as potentially a gastric abnormality. On the other hand, bowel movements of normal frequency are no guarantee of bowel normalcy.

What should "normal" stool look like? Would you believe that it took the medical community until *1990* before someone first addressed this question in a formal matter? In that year, some enterprising researchers at the University of Bristol in the United Kingdom came up with what is now referred to as the Bristol Stool Form Scale to categorize various stool forms. They devised a seven-point scale in which stools were scored according to cohesion and surface cracking as follows: 1, separate hard lumps like nuts; 2, sausage shaped but lumpy; 3, like a sausage or snake but with cracks on its surface; 4, like a sausage or snake, smooth and soft; 5, soft blobs with clear cut edges; 6, fluffy pieces with ragged edges, a mushy stool; and 7, watery, no solid pieces. Some of the tests they performed were on patients with irritable bowel syndrome, where they were able to inverse correlate the stool scale number with actual whole gut transit time, where the lower the number the longer the transit time [19]. This data is difficult to interpret because of the varied diets of the participants. Further studies have inverse related gut transit time with dietary fiber, which can be controlled by fruit consumption.

Ah, but we do have more clues from MA. There is no toilet paper in the animal kingdom! Yes, chimps have been known to use leaves for occasional anal wiping (usually a sign of toxicity), and some species are famous for doing that for each other. However, by and large, there is no need for anal wiping because the form and consistency of their stool is such that there is no significant residue. Enter toilet paper.

Apparently, toilet paper was used in China as early as 900 A.D., but that's like a minute ago on the human timeline. Even more recently, in step with the nineteenth century advent of the toilet, flat sheet paper, and then roll paper, came of age. Before that, people used newsprint or mail order catalogues, and before that they used their hand (left or right depending on culture), and some still do. This to me serves as a clue as to how our stool should shape up. We should not need toilet paper, which is probably one of the first things we would grab in case of an evacuation. The fact that we need toilet paper to wipe away residue is testimony to our dietary detour and the resultant ill health of our gut. Referring back to the Bristol Scale, categories 1-4 qualify for leaving no or minimal residue. Category 1, however, is clearly a case of constipation and is usually accompanied with straining, eventually leading to hemorrhoids, hardly part of MA's plan.

So, from my analysis, a normal stool should be sausage shaped, varying from a rough to a smooth exterior, eliminated without straining and occurring at least once a day. As you may remember, toilet paper was on my list of Faulty Human Trials in Table 1. It seems to me that the mere fact that it is in such widespread use is clear evidence that our bowel movements are unnatural. Further, the use of toilet paper has conditioned us to accept this state of affairs, and to pay little or no attention to what is in the toilet bowl, allowing gut problems to go unnoticed for years, if not a lifetime.

Next on the stool list is the age-old question of floaters versus sinkers. As discussed earlier in the section on bile salts, floating stools can be a sign of excessive fat content, symptoms of maldigestion that may be related to the gall bladder. A second reason for floating stools is excessive trapped gas, also a sign of maldigestion. So, the winners are the sinkers.

Moving on to color, the foods we eat can have a dramatic effect on stool color. In *The Original Diet*, the types of fruits eaten may affect stool color, particularly those with high carotenoid (orange) content. Typically, stool color is a dark brown. Green or yellow (bile color) may indicate excessive bile in the stool, usually from very fast transit time, not allowing for bile recycling in the small intestine. Normally, only about 5% of the circulating bile is excreted. Pale stool color, such as grey or whitish, may well be a sign of insufficient bile, and the use of bile salt supplements might be a good idea. If you find during detoxification that your stool tends toward numbers 5-7 on the Bristol scale, your colon may not be removing and recycling sufficient water, leading toward dehydration. One idea is to drink a large glass of water after every bowel movement.

Finally, strong stool odor is a sure sign of maldigestion, whereby undigested food is being excreted, and strong odors would not have been amenable to survival in PA's environment. Rodale found that taking dolomite could reduce stool odor, indicating that it has a strong effect on normalizing digestion [10]. This completes the description of stool, and here is a concise summary: the goal is soft, sinking, sienna, stinkless sausages. Now, onward to clues from MA on how to defecate.

From studies of indigenous societies and animals, we know that the natural way to defecate is to squat—not to sit—and in much of the undeveloped world, squatting is still very much the norm. It was less than 150 years ago, in the latter part of the nineteenth century that the toilet arrived on the scene and slowly changed the style of how most of us learned to defecate. What has the toilet revolution wrought? Some studies show that the colon actually lines up more effectively in a squatting position, and that, in theory, you get a more relaxed and thorough bowel movement. The long-term benefits may include less stress and strain on the intestinal and urinary tracts, more complete elimination, and other benefits yet to be determined. Some keen-eyed medical observers over the years have noted that many different bowel, bladder, and pelvic conditions, previously rare or unknown, suddenly became commonplace in the Western world in the last half of the nineteenth century. Their observations suggest that by returning to squatting, as MA intended, we may eliminate problems such as hemorrhoids.

If you are interested in experimenting with the concept of squatting to line up your colon naturally, the least expensive method is to elevate your feet, say, about eight to ten inches from the floor using books or bricks, while sitting on the toilet. A more elegant solution is to purchase one of the many devices for this purpose, which I affectionately call "stool stools" [20]. These devices put you in a squatting position as you lean forward, and it doesn't take long before you feel very comfortable and natural with it, so much so that when you're traveling and you don't have it, you feel like something's wrong. This issue may seem somewhat humorous because we have all grown up on the toilet, so to speak. However, it's really just another example of how we have deviated from what MA intended with unknown consequences simply because of our arrogance in thinking we know what we're doing. Children are potty trained, but it may well be that adults need to be potty retrained.

It has been my experience that deviations from the ideal in the realm of defecation result from diet and detox issues, and a goal of The Wellness Project is to restore order to the gut. This accomplishes two purposes: first, it will improve nutrient absorption, and second, it will maximize the use of the defecation pathway for toxin removal. The dirt components of the diet, such as spore-forming bacteria, can be instrumental in restoring bowel movements to normal by providing the right mix of bowel flora.

I want to make it clear that I am not saying everyone has to meet The Detox Plan BM criteria to be healthy. I have no doubt that there are people out there who can have two messy BMs per month and lead a very long and healthy life. Probably these same folks can thrive on cake and soda, and are the *winners* for the moment. I doubt they are reading this book.

Breathing

Breathing gets rid of toxic chemicals through gas exchange in our lungs, where we take in oxygen and expel gaseous wastes. While we can promote that process with breathing techniques that can be learned as part of some yoga and meditation practices, there are additional ways to enhance this detox pathway. Deep breathing requires unrestricted movement of the belly, ribcage, and diaphragm. Enter tight clothing.

I'm not going to suggest you walk around with a loincloth but there are some lessons to be learned from Flintstone® fashions. One would assume that hunter-gatherers figured out how to clothe themselves using the skins of animals. Whatever they wore would have been minimal and it would have been loose, whereas today (except for baggy-panted juveniles) we tend toward the tight in order to show off buns, boobs, and biceps. What's the difference between loose and tight? Studies have shown that tight clothing does affect both the anatomy and physiology in ways that may be detrimental to health. One example is brassieres.

Indigenous women did not wear them, but throughout recent history, women have used a variety of garments and devices to cover, restrain, or elevate their breasts. From the sixteenth century onwards, the corset hoisted the breasts of wealthier women. Then, in the latter part of the nineteenth century, clothing designers began experimenting with alternatives that by the early twentieth century had morphed into what we now recognize as contemporary bras and a multi-billion-dollar industry. The emphasis has pretty much shifted from functionality to fashion, with an underlying assumption throughout this evolutionary process that no harm is being done.

However, at least one set of studies I am aware of has investigated the possibility that brassieres may contribute to the incidence of breast cancer. These studies were featured in a widely publicized 1995 book entitled *Dressed to Kill* [21]. The authors collected striking evidence directly correlating the number of hours per day a woman wears a bra with the risk of breast cancer. Women who wear tight-fitting bras 24 hours a day are 125 times more likely to have breast cancer than women who do not wear bras at all. One theory behind this correlation is that bras may be constricting the flow of lymph from the breast area, and restricting the flow of lymph into the axillary lymph nodes under each arm. As I mentioned earlier, the lymph system is poorly understood, but it is a major system within the body for transporting toxins and getting them into the blood stream for evacuation. To the extent that process is interfered with, it may contribute to toxin accumulation in the breast. See the side box entitled HealthBra™ for a short description of my efforts in this area.

For those female readers wanting to experiment, not wearing brassieres is clearly what MA intended. Other than that, it would seem prudent to wear them as loose as possible, for the shortest time possible, and as unstructured as possible (perhaps without an underwire, which usually can be removed with a scissor). If you can see indentions in your skin upon removal, this may be a clue that your bra is indeed causing restriction of some sort, such as lymph or blood flow or the ability to take full deep breaths, none of which is a good idea. Some companies have produced bras designed to include lymph massage as a feature [22].

As tight bras are to women, tight briefs may be to men. Researchers have found that they hold a man's testicles close to the body and raise the temperature of the sperm. This decreases its lifespan and could affect fertility. In some problem infertility cases, men have been asked to switch to loose-fitting boxers. Guys, take this as a clue from MA – loosen up. Is there a difference between wearing a belt or suspenders? It seems logical that constricting the abdomen with a tight belt for many hours a day could adversely affect abdominal blood flow and the digestive system, as well as the ability to take deep breaths. Avoiding tight belts and pants are among the lifestyle changes suggested by some doctors to overweight patients with heartburn issues.

HealthBra™

A disturbing incidence of breast cancer in prior generations in my family inspired me to suggest to my wife and daughters that they abandon their brassieres. The suggestion was not well received, so I set out to design bras that would minimize the restriction of lymph flow. I eventually created a variety of designs with the help of some product designers, and patented them (US Patents Nos. 6,086,450 and 6,361,397). In my conversations with the authors of *Dressed to Kill*, they predicted there would be little interest from the undergarment industry to produce products of this kind, and the authors themselves had been threatened with a lawsuit when they were about to publish their book. One could imagine the difficulty of a brassiere manufacturer producing a bra that is designed to overcome what might be negative health effects of their previous designs. I remain optimistic that this area will ultimately get the attention it deserves.

Bad breath may be another sign from MA that you are excreting bad stuff through your lungs. Faulty diet, and/or toxins from bad dentition and gum problems, or from gut backup or throat infections, can all cause it. Below, I will discuss the use of clay to absorb a lot of this junk during the detox process, and the use of spore-formers to get rid of putrid gut bacteria. The breath should be sweet day and night in a healthy body.

Sweating

Sweating has proven to be a major detoxification pathway for a variety of reasons. First, the large surface area of the skin enables significant amounts of sweat to push or carry toxins to the surface along short, direct pathways from virtually any part of the body. Second, unlike urination and defecation, we have some control over when and how much we sweat, leading to a detoxification program that can be scheduled. Third, it bypasses the digestive system, which in many cases is not functioning properly because of the toxic load. That is not to say, however, that toxins do not interfere with the ability to sweat, which I can attest to personally. As an example, magnesium deficiency, caused by many toxins, can suppress normal sweating.

The easiest way to promote sweating is to heat the body. One way is through the natural fever we develop when ill, which is certainly a clue from MA and should never be suppressed unless necessary to prevent brain damage. A more pleasant way to sweat naturally (at least for some) is through exercise, and in fact, I consider sweating as a major health benefit of exercise. Yet another way is artificially to heat the body with an external source, such as a sauna. I will be going into this topic in some depth in the next section, as external heat is an extremely important detoxification tool.

This brings me to the subject of antiperspirants. Using antiperspirants is really fooling with MA on several counts. First, it is suppressing the very mechanism we so heavily depend upon to excrete toxins. There are large sweat and lymph glands under the arms—major detoxification pathways and outlets near the heart and lungs critical to keeping the body clean. Antiperspirants interfere with their natural function. Second, the chemicals used to create these products are themselves toxic and usually include aluminum and possibly zirconium. Applying aluminum under the arms (and with women, it's often freshly shaved underarms) is really not a good idea since it can be absorbed in large amounts, further toxifying the body. Aluminum is believed to be a neurotoxin and has been implicated as a possible cause in Alzheimer's disease, so daily use of an antiperspirant could contribute to a dreaded disease [23]. To absorb sweat, consider pads of some sort. I will also discuss below the use of clay and magnesium as other alternatives.

Regarding deodorants, if you have extreme body odor, that is likely an indication of improper diet and/or significant toxins. Remember that a strong body odor is not conducive to survival in the wild, as it attracts predators, another clue from MA. Because sweating is a natural detoxification pathway, food odors passed through the skin may well be a sign that you are eating the wrong stuff. We can all remember being around others reeking of garlic and onions (plant bulbs not on *The Original Diet*), and this may actually be a smelly clue from MA to leave her bulbs alone. So, if you smell like dinner, you probably ate the wrong food, and your body is trying to get rid of it. Many in the medical field dismiss body odor as simply a normal bacterial decay process, but they have nothing with which to compare it. The word *normal* has no real meaning unless you can compare it to some *baseline*, which is a major goal of *The Wellness Project.*

Having said all that about odors, I feel compelled to tell you about a natural body deodorizer – magnesium! Buried in the archives of early magnesium research are some fascinating experiments and observations showing that taking sufficient magnesium supplementation (actually, dolomite was used in the studies) completely eliminated underarm, body, urine, stool, and foot odor [10]. I am not aware of any studies to determine why magnesium acts in this manner, but it surely points to a detox effect of some sort. As readers know by now, I am not shy about speculating, so here is something to ponder. Many of us have heard the expression "the smell of fear," which is loosely defined as an odor emanating from an animal or person in a highly fearful situation. Well, magnesium is quickly excreted when we are under stress, so could the origin of this expression be the depletion of magnesium (resulting in body odor) as a result of extreme stress (fear)?

Chapter 5 - Natural Detoxification Agents

This section is a discussion of some of the more important detoxifying agents that would have been easily accessible to PA, with the exception of a sauna, which is a modern day substitute for PA running around in the tropical sun with few clothes on.

Sauna

Sauna is a Finnish word for a small room or house in which one can experience dry or wet heat sessions. Indigenous tribes have used sweat lodges for a very long time as a ritual means of cleansing through sweating. The wet sauna uses various methods to produce steam, resulting in a humid environment with air temperatures in the range of

175-200 degrees F. Unless purified water is used to produce the steam, it is possible to inhale and absorb toxins such as chlorine or fluoride, much like the shower situation, and fungus growth is another possible issue. The closest analogy I can think of to a wet sauna in nature would be hot mineral springs, which can be quite healing.

The modern dry sauna is called the FIR (far infrared) sauna, and is one of my favorite detoxification tools. It is well known that the human body radiates infrared (IR) energy at a wavelength of about 10 microns, well within the warming portion of the spectrum of sunlight. The idea behind FIR sauna is to generate IR energy in a range of wavelengths near this value in a sauna environment. There is much anecdotal information on the detoxification benefits of FIR vs. wet sauna, mixed in with a lot of marketing hype. I and others with whom I have consulted have found saunas to be of great benefit in promoting the excretion of a variety of toxins, from heavy metals to pesticides to prescription and recreational drugs. Some excellent books on the subject are *Sauna Therapy* by Lawrence Wilson, and *The Holistic Handbook of Sauna Therapy* by Nenah Sylver [24] [25]. How do we know it works? Well, personally, I can see it in my skin, which for most of my life has been my visual indicator of toxicity. My observations, in conjunction with the pioneering work of Paul Dantzig into the cutaneous signs of mercury poisoning, provided me with a handy way of evaluating progress in my own mercury detoxification program, and I could track it as a function of sauna use [26-30] [31]. I also feel better than usual when I use the sauna regularly. Since the mantra of the dermatology community is "name it, we tame it," I will take this opportunity to hereby name the constellation of undiagnosed skin manifestations due to mercury toxicity as *Mercuroderma*!

Although quite controversial because of its ties to a religious organization, the Narconon program of drug rehabilitation has apparently been successful in using sauna treatment to sweat out drugs. More recently, a similar program was used to treat New York City firefighters exposed to a wide range of toxins in the 9/11 debacle, with reported successes. There are anecdotal stories of past drug users reliving "highs" during sessions, and still others report seeing and smelling various substances in their sweat that they remember taking decades ago. The bottom line for me is that I intend to use my sauna regularly for life in an effort to keep up with the unavoidable toxic load in today's world. With some caveats, the concept seems to fit well within the natural experience of being exposed to the warming rays of sunlight, and it actually feels that way. Unlike the wet variety, the FIR sauna has a lower air temperature, in the 90-120 degree F range, so it is much more comfortable, and the lack of use of water eliminates problems such as chlorine and fungal contamination.

It is helpful to put the FIR sauna experience in perspective with respect to nature. The FIR frequency spectrum is within that of normal sunlight, and the air temperatures are within the range one might find in the summer in some desert resorts such as Palm Springs and Scottsdale, or tropical locales. Actually, if you live in or have access to these locations, you could start a detox program simply by sitting outside wearing minimal clothing in an area receiving sunlight energy, directly or indirectly. If not, here are some suggestions in purchasing an FIR sauna.

There are many FIR sauna manufacturers, some reputable and some not. My preference is one built of wood, using a species (at least on the inside) such as poplar or alder that has minimal outgassing of volatile compounds. Many on the market have an interior made of cedar, which outgases terpines that may be irritating to some people. The sauna should have a large complement of ceramic FIR emitters, and a temperature control. One brand that has a good reputation is Thermal Life made by High Tech Health [32].

Less expensive models, called cabinets, wrap around the body, leaving the head exposed, and for some people, this is more comfortable. It may also have an advantage if there are medical or dental problems requiring avoidance of heating the head (the issue of dental amalgams is discussed in a later section). One concern I have about some of the cabinets is their use of plastic for the enclosure, since the elevated temperatures of the unit may well cause these plastics to outgas toxins that are absorbed or inhaled by the user. For another option, you can inexpensively build your own sauna in an area as small as a closet, as described in the Wilson book cited above [24]. Here are some sauna protocols.

Sauna therapy, like any other form of detoxification, can cause a die-off reaction as described above, and may be harmful to those with specific medical conditions or implants. For this reason, begin by using the sauna in a very slow, low dose manner. There is actually some controversy as to the harmful effects of sauna, and there are rare reports of cases of toxic individuals who seem to get worse, but this is no different from possible responses to most of the other detox protocols. I encourage anyone with a serious medical condition or taking a lot of medications who would like to begin sauna therapy to read Larry Wilson's book on the subject, and perhaps consult with him [33] or others with experience in the field. Two that come to mind are Dr. Dietrich Klinghardt [34], and Dr. Hans Gruenn [35], both of whom use sauna therapy in their detox practices. In any event, at the beginning, it might be prudent to have a buddy along to monitor you during sessions.

I would also suggest reading the section below on alkalinity, since I believe it can enhance all detox protocols, including sauna. Finally and most important, note that body stores of magnesium (and other minerals) are depleted as a result of elevated body temperature and sweating. Therefore, I encourage sauna beginners to first test their magnesium levels and begin a supplement program if needed. Interestingly, there is some anecdotal evidence that magnesium supports sweating, so perhaps an inability to sweat is a marker for magnesium deficiency.

Along my journey in the world of sauna therapy, I was fortunate to have Dr. Wilson as a coach to coax me along as I got started. Knowing I was mercury toxic, with the usual attendant hypo-metabolic issues, including the inability to sweat very much, I began very cautiously, and I would encourage others to do the same. I used the low temperature setting (about 90 degrees F), and started with only a five-minute session time once every other day. After a month, I went to daily sessions and began to notice an increase in sweating (I was also supplementing with magnesium). I slowly raised the temperature and increased the session time to 20 minutes, and now (several years later) I enjoy the 120 degree F setting and sweat quite profusely. It is important to replenish water and minerals (particularly magnesium and potassium) after each session, using the protocols described above. Doing so insufficiently is very likely to be quite unpleasant, particularly if you experience muscle cramping. After each session, I suggest quickly showering in warm water to wash off the toxins, and not reusing (or sharing) towels until they have been washed.

While we are on the topic of washing clothes, how about a soap derived from fruit? The fruit from the Chinese Soapberry tree (Sapindus Mukorossi), referred to as a soap nut, is very high in saponins, a natural detergent, and makes a soap for washing clothing and other items. It is supplied in its natural nut form [36], in powder form [37], and as a liquid [38]. It is hypoallergenic and biodegradable, with many uses.

In an FIR sauna, you are surrounded by electrical wiring, which can subject the body to a substantial electrical field. This can easily be measured using a digital AC millivoltmeter connected between an electrical ground terminal and your body. I have measured voltages as high as 8 volts AC on my body in the sauna, and although I do not know what effect this may have on the detox process, this electrical field induced charge is quite easy and inexpensive to eliminate. In the section below entitled the EMF (Electromagnetic Field) Problem I go into some depth regarding the potential advantages of keeping our bodies in electrical contact with the earth. It is there that I will show examples of how to do so, even in the sauna. Because I have adopted sauna therapy as a part of my lifestyle, I built my house to include a room devoted to detoxification, including the sauna, a system for connecting myself to earth ground, a connection to the house music system, and both a filtered mineral water spout and shower just outside the sauna. I feel it is important to make taking a sauna a fun experience that you can look forward to, either alone or with others.

Before leaving the sauna discussion, I want to mention some products that are also based on the use of FIR energy, and that have proved quite useful in treating chronic detox symptoms and pain in general. They are FIR heating pads that can be used locally to deliver FIR energy to specific parts of the body. The purpose of these devices is not to cause sweating, but to create healing effects which result either through the heat itself or the particular wavelength, or from reasons we have yet to discover. The brand I use is *Thermotex*, and the pads come in a variety of sizes [39]. Their successful use with horses and other animals prompted my wife and me to acquire one designed as a pet bed, and our cats love it. My personal theory is that, for indoor pets, it recreates the natural experience of lying on warm earth heated by sunlight. If you use an FIR pad, I have found it helpful to be aware of the possibility of referred pain while detoxing, where your neck pain may be due, for example, to toxins accumulating in the gut. So, experiment with the pad to see what areas of the body work best. It may be that using the pad on the abdomen will alleviate neck pain. In other words, do not assume that the origin of the pain is the part that is hurting.

Alkalinity

Those readers familiar with detoxification may be puzzled by the inclusion of alkalinity as a detox protocol, but from my research, it is an important factor, without which many conventional detox protocols will not work, or will work poorly. As many of you know, acidity and alkalinity are conveniently measured using a pH scale, where values from 0-7 are considered acidic, and from 7-14 are considered alkaline (the value 7 is considered neutral).

My research on this subject actually took shape when investigating how heavy metals such as mercury, lead, and cadmium are dealt with by MA in the outside world. The results were somewhat astonishing, and had to do with dirt and pH. It is well known that humic and fulvic acids in the soil can act as heavy metal scavengers, adsorbing and transporting them. Adsorption occurs when a substance, such as a heavy metal, forms one or more of several types of bonds with the surface of an adsorbing material such as the soil acid matrix. This is as opposed to absorption, where two substances diffuse into each other to form a solution.

It is also known that the soil acids have the capability of desorbing the metals, or dropping them from the fulvic/humic acid matrix [40]. Much research has been performed on these issues, because heavy metal sequestration is an important issue in toxic site remediation [41]. Several factors enter into the desorption phenomenon, but the one that caught my attention was that an increase in pH vastly increased the strength of attachment between the soil acid matrix and the metals. Conversely, at low (acidic) pH values, the soil acid matrix lets go of the metals. The same scenario takes place when clay, fulvic/humic acids, and heavy metals were mixed together [41].

The reason that pH caught my eye is that it had come to my attention before in my research into spore-forming bacteria, discussed below. Remarkably, spore-formers also have the ability to bond with heavy metals via adsorption, and they too can release the metals under certain conditions, including low pH (an acidic environment) [42] [43] [44]. So, now we have three elements of soil that I consider important to health (humic/fulvic acids, spore-forming bacteria, and clay), all capable of binding with heavy (and other) metals, where the pH of the mix is a determinant as to the strength of the soil-metal bond, and hence whether the soil will hold onto the metals or release them. This adsorption/desorption characteristic is actually used by environmental scientists for toxic cleanup. For example, soil bacteria, also called biomass, can be used to grab toxic metals at a high pH level, and then made to let go of them at an appropriate reclamation site by lowering the pH. Thus, the metals get to be recycled into industry, and the biomass can be reused again for toxic cleanup by re-alkalization.

You may ask what all of this has to do with human detoxification. I am conducting a personal detoxification study, which I call the Dirt Detox protocol™, detailed more thoroughly in the next section on dirt, in which the pH of urine plays a critical role. For this section, I will concentrate on ways in which one can measure and adjust urine pH. There are no end of books and supplements devoted to body alkaline/acid balance, many of which seem to contradict each other, but there is general agreement among authors that diet has an impact, with fruits and some vegetables (not seeds) having an alkalizing effect. In *The Original Diet*, fruit, mineral water, and dolomite act as natural alkaline balancers.

During detoxification of heavy metals, particularly in the case of mercury detox, I and others have found it difficult to keep urine pH in balance (it tends to be too acid) without some supplement help. This is important because it has been shown that alkaline urine promotes the excretion of mercury [4]. The first step is to get some pH paper to measure your urine. I use pHydrion brand pH sticks with a pH range of 5.0 to 9.0, or their pH paper in roll form with a range of 5.5 to 8.0 [45]. The objective is to measure urine pH a few times per day, with the goal of keeping it neutral or higher, say between 7 and 8.

In addition to the natural alkalizing agents of fruit, mineral water, and dolomite (calcium and magnesium carbonates), there are two supplement categories that have been used to alkalize urine pH. The first are mineral citrates such as potassium citrate, which may be taken with or without meals. I experiment with the dose until I find the minimum that keeps urine pH above 7 for most of the day when detoxifying heavy metals [46] [47]. Those taking drugs or those who have kidney issues need to monitor potassium levels (preferably red blood cell levels) while taking potassium supplements.

Another alkalizing approach is to use bicarbonates such as potassium and/or sodium bicarbonate (baking soda). There are many alkalizing bicarbonates on the market, and they should not be taken with meals because they tend to neutralize stomach acid, interfering with proper digestion. My preference is to use additional mineral citrates to achieve daytime alkaline urine when detoxing heavy metals. Alka-Seltzer® Gold is one example of a commercial product that provides sodium and potassium citrates. On the days when not detoxing heavy metals, I do not take supplements to alkalize urine, and let my body establish its own acid/alkaline balance. The subject of alkalinity will be further discussed in the experimental Dirt Detox Protocol™ below.

Dirt

By dirt, I mean soil, but the word dirt is so much more dramatic! Few people appreciate the fact that soil itself is a form of food. It is unlikely that PA washed off what she/he ate, and so ingested some soil with fruit, animal prey, and drinking water. Surprisingly, soil contains many beneficial bacteria, amino acids, and trace minerals, as well as other compounds that we have yet to identify. From my research, there appear to be four separate groups of soil materials that contribute to health both for animals (including humans), and plants.

The first group is in the form of acids named fulvic and humic acids, which are major constituents of what you may be familiar with as potting soil, humus, or peat moss. This material is the accumulation of partially decayed vegetable matter, before it turns into coal or oil. It is great for plant growth, and some interesting research has been conducted regarding the beneficial effects from human consumption [48]. What becomes clear from this research is the importance of starting with very clean soil, free of toxins. Put another way, if you ingest toxic soil, it will toxify you, which appears to have happened on at least some occasions

[49]. My approach was to find suppliers who have been providing these soil components as supplements for human consumption for a decade or more. In the U.S., the predominant source of soil for these supplements is known as the Fruitland Formation, located in Northwestern New Mexico. This shale formation from which the soil is taken is the remains of an ancient shallow fresh-water sea dating from about 80 million years ago. Several companies have been mining the soil from it for decades for use as soil conditioners as well as for animal and human use [50] [51]. Some of the cited human benefits include improved mineral utilization, and antiviral properties. These soil acids also bind with heavy metals so they can pass out of the body, and act as an immune system stimulant.

One of several companies that have been offering soil products for human use for some time is Morningstar Minerals [52], who offer capsules and liquids containing high concentrations of fulvic and humic acids. The products I use are those with minimal processing, referred to as Immune Boost 77 (capsules) and Vitality Boost HA (liquid). It seems to me that PA would have ingested a daily dose of these acids by drinking water found in tree and rock depressions, and even in flowing stream water that picks up soil along the way. I add one capsule or one ounce of the liquid each day to my drinking water as a way of more closely duplicating PA's diet. There is a more thorough discussion of humic and fulvic acids below. Note that the high carbon content of these supplements may cause darkening of the water and the stool.

The second group of materials from soil is bacteria, and they turn out to be an important component of Nature's Detox Plan. These bacteria, sometimes inaccurately referred to as soil based organisms (SBOs), are quite different from the conventional probiotics most of us are familiar with, such as acidophilus, so to avoid confusion I will not refer to them as probiotics. While these organisms are certainly found in great quantity in soil, it really is not clear where they might have originated. In addition to soil, they are found throughout nature in water, dust, air, and in the intestines of animals, insects, and sea life, but they are not native to the human gut and do not take up permanent residence there, unlike conventional probiotics. They survive stomach acid, thrive in an oxygen environment, have the ability to form spores (actually endospores) and can bind with toxins.

The ability to form spores has resulted in the name *spore-formers* being used to describe these bacteria, and I will refer to them as such. I will be going into some detail in this section because I believe they are a very important missing ingredient in our diets that can have a profound positive effect on our health. Some of the reasons they are missing include the widespread use of fungicides and pesticides in the soil, and the use of disinfectants such as chlorine in our water supplies, all of which can prevent spore-formers from proliferating.

There is research being performed on spore-formers in the belief that they may eventually replace conventional antibiotics, which are rapidly becoming obsolete due to bacterial resistance. Spore-formers could have appeared in PA's diet from dirt or dust on fruit, in drinking water, and from the intestinal contents of their animal prey, discussed in the probiotics section below.

For some of my comments, I will be drawing from an excellent review of the subject entitled *The Use of Bacterial Spore Formers as Probiotics* by H. Hong, et al. [53]. One simplified way to understand spore-forming bacteria is to use a seed analogy. Just like a plant seed that has a strong coating protecting the embryo, the spore-formers have a strong coating protecting an endospore. They can lie dormant for years until germinated by being placed in a suitable environment, which usually includes a liquid. The human gut is an ideal environment for many of these species to germinate. I like to think of the spore-formers as MA's way of providing us with "friendly seeds" designed to grow for a short time in the "soil" of our intestines and provide great health benefits. Having said that, there are spore-formers that are quite nasty, such as anthrax, so it behooves us to tread with care in this area.

Although research is still in its infancy as it applies to humans, the potential benefits that can be derived from these bacteria are somewhat overwhelming. From what is known, immune system stimulation and the generation of unique antimicrobials are just two areas of great interest. A third benefit is that of competitive exclusion (CE), where the spore-formers take up temporary residence, and through a variety of poorly understood mechanisms, exclude pathogens from adhering to the gut wall. At one time, I thought that conventional probiotics could fill this role, but from my experience, they cannot hold a candle to the spore-formers in the pathogen exclusion arena. Yet another area of interest for spore-formers is that of cardiovascular disease. A fermented soy product called natto (and nattokinase) has been touted as preventing heart attacks and cancer, among other benefits. Well, natto is made by fermenting soy with bacillus subtilis, a spore-former, so it is certainly possible that it is the subtilis, not the soy, which is responsible for the benefits.

Reading between the lines of some of the research studies [54], I ponder the following. If ingesting a somewhat continuous supply of spore-formers with our food (they tend to last less than 30 days in the human gut) can effectively exclude pathogens from taking up residence, could they be a preventive for a whole host of bad guys such as salmonella, C. difficile, H. pylori, MRSA, anthrax, and the bacteria responsible for malaria and Lyme disease? In the fungal arena, there is a great deal of evidence that spore-formers can exclude Candida and other fungi from the gut and this will be covered in more depth below. Spore-formers are also known bioinsecticides, opening up a fertile area of research into a natural form of mosquito control [55]. By now, you may be sensing a great deal of excitement on my part for the goodies described in this dirt section.

Here is how I use spore-formers as part of the detox program. My approach, as in the case of the humic and fulvic acid products, is to find suppliers that have been providing spore-formers for human use for a decade or more. Several species of the *bacillus* genus of spore formers have seen extensive use in human supplements worldwide, and they include b. subtilis, b. licheniformis, b. megaterium, b. clausii, b. coagulans, and b. laterosporus. After some research, I have chosen two species that have a long history of non-pathogenic use and favorable symptom relief. The first is bacillus coagulans, which is also called (somewhat incorrectly) lactobacillus sporogenes. It is supplied as capsules under the lactobacillus sporogenes name by both Thorne Research [56] and Pure Encapsulations [57]. The second species is bacillus laterosporus, strain BOD [58], which is widely distributed by O'Donnell Formulas under the names Flora Balance and Latero-Flora as capsules and powder. These supplements can be purchased at many supplement retailers [59]. Because they are found in soil and water in their natural environment, I take them with drinking water along with the humic-fulvic acid supplements. For a maintenance dose, I use one capsule per day, or an equivalent dose of the powder.

Although not a normal dietary component, other very valuable forms of dirt -known as clays- have always been used in the animal kingdom and among humans as a detoxifying agent, and form the third group of materials that make up dirt. I have devoted an entire section to the health benefits of clay below. As you will see in that discussion, before cooking allowed PA to experiment with eating plants that are toxic when raw, if it was necessary to eat these foods or face starvation, PA sought out certain clays to eat with the food. These acted to either adsorb or otherwise detoxify the toxic compounds in the plant food. We, too, can use clay to assist in removing a variety of other toxins from our body.

The fourth component of dirt for purposes of our discussion is dolomite, which was discussed in the section on water. Dolomite, a rock that is a form of limestone, is widely found on and in the Earth's surface as stone formations and as natural sediment in the soil. It is discussed further in the mineral section below.

In summary, there are four components to dirt as it is defined for the Original Detox Plan: humic/fulvic acids, spore-forming bacteria, clay, and dolomite. We will visit each in the following sections.

Clay

Would you walk miles through the jungle to get to a particular type of dirt that you then proceed to eat in great quantity? Well, many animals (including humans) do so, for reasons that are still unfolding. The dirt types they are seeking are generally referred to as clays, one of MA's secret weapons in the game of survival. It is not fully understood how clay-eating interacts with animals, but several theories have been put forward. The six explanations most discussed among zoologists, anthropologists, and doctors are to assuage hunger, to provide grit for grinding food in the stomach, to buffer stomach contents, to cure diarrhea, to serve as a mineral supplement, and to adsorb toxins [60].

We are going to discuss the last regarding excluded plant foods, the main reason for avoiding them being the load of natural toxins they contain. While we in the Western world are fortunate that we have available to us year round healthy foods, our Paleo ancestors were not so fortunate. It is easy to image how, for a variety of environmental reasons, a shortage in animal food periodically could have occurred in the Paleo era. In such a case, PA might have had to resort to foods that are normally toxic, as a survival strategy. Enter clay.

Humans ate clay to protect themselves against these food toxins. For example, modernly, some South American Indians regularly dine on bitter, toxic wild potatoes containing a nasty alkaloid that by itself would cause stomach pains and vomiting. However, the Indians have learned to make the potatoes safe and palatable by eating them with an alkaloid-binding clay. California Indians and natives of Sardinia used to make a bread from nutritious acorns whose sole drawback was that they contained bitter, astringent, and toxic tannic acid. Both the Indians and the Sardinians mixed the acorn flour with a clay that reduced tannic acid by up to 77 percent. These peoples did not understand alkaloid chemistry or adsorption, but they did discover empirically that eating clay made these foods edible and thus avoided starvation. Wild animals and birds worldwide do the same thing, and are able to consume plants with potent toxins such as strychnine [61]. I am certainly not advocating eating toxic foods on a *regular* basis, relying on clay to clean up the toxins. Not enough is known about the types and amounts of clay to be used for a given toxic food. Further, whenever available, animals eat their native foods and only deviate when necessary. I intend to follow that example.

Returning to some of the other explanations for eating clay, some clays are believed to act as mineral supplements as well as immune system boosters in ways we do not fully understand. Pregnant and lactating women in indigenous regions are known to crave soil, consuming more than an ounce per day. Clay in the form of kaolin was used for many years in the preparation Kaopectate® to ameliorate diarrhea, and supposedly was removed from the product because of some form of contamination. We will cover the clay contamination issue below. Regarding assuaging hunger, the Ottomac Indians of South America made soil balls six inches in diameter and ate more than one pound per day during the flood season when it was difficult to find food, and clay eating has also been reported in Western Europe during famines. In this detox section, we are going to make use of several of these clay characteristics. Unfortunately, as in many of the other fields we have traversed, little research has been done in the area of clay as it relates to human health (there is no money in it), while there are a wealth of studies on its use in water treatment and other toxic abatement applications.

Beginning with the adsorption of toxins, anecdotal evidence abounds in the curative properties of clay with respect to toxin removal [62] [63] [64, 65] [66], and a website dedicated to the healing applications of clay, created by Jason Eaton, has a wealth of information on the subject [67]. Because *The Original Diet* removes virtually all natural toxins, this enables clay to be used as necessary in detox protocols to remove modern toxins such as heavy metals, pesticides, parasites, and bacteria. Here are a few caveats. Since we don't know for sure what is adsorbed and what is not, it is prudent to make sure we take clay an hour or more before or after taking food or detox supplements or medications. Second, it is imperative that the clay material we start with is clean (devoid of toxins), to prevent unintentionally toxifying ourselves with "dirty clay." Regarding toxins in clay, they naturally contain aluminum hydroxide and iron, but eons of use have demonstrated that neither produces an excess of aluminum or iron in the body. Third, clay only works if it is hydrated, that is, mixed with water. So taking clay if you are dehydrated is unproductive and could be dangerous by allowing the formation of a blockage in the gut. Clay should always be taken with water, or dissolved in saliva before swallowing.

Here are my suggestions for ingesting clay as a detox agent. I plan to use clay as part of a lifetime detoxification regimen on the basis that we are continuously exposed to environmental toxins. The widespread use of clay for millennia in the animal world is a good enough "clinical trial" for me. I have used and evaluated three U.S. sources of clay. Two are considered to be calcium-bentonite types (also referred to as Montmorillonite), and the third is a sodium-bentonite type. These three are all from the smectite family of clays that have been found overall to have the most favorable healing characteristics. There are hundreds of other types from various parts of the world, all with their unique following. The first source is called Pascalite clay [68], and is available as a powder or in capsules for ingestion. The second source is called Terramin [69], and is available as powder and tablets for ingestion. The third, Redmond clay, which is the sodium-bentonite clay, is only available in powder form [70]. All of the companies referenced have an excellent reputation and have been supplying clean clay for many years. As far as which brand is best for you personally to use, I know of no other way to determine this except by experiment.

How you ingest the clay depends on several factors, the first of which is whether you like the taste of clay (I do). If you do not, the choices are to take it as capsules or tablets. For a short term detox dosing schedule of five days every two weeks, I take two capsules or tablets or a half-teaspoon of the powder upon arising and at bedtime. I am sure to drink at least 8 ounces of water with them. As reported in the literature, you may see a wide range of symptom relief from eating clay, including digestive, skin, pain, and mental clarity areas, all pointing to a reduction in toxic load.

Some people are distressed by the prospect of eating clay, and for them we have the art of pelotherapy, the topical use of dirt, covering everything from mudpacks to medical poultices to clay baths. Both Pascalite and Terramin brands also sell topical preparations for use in various applications, some pre-prepared. The references cited above will provide a lot of information on the topical use of clays, some of which seem to border on the miraculous, including curing somewhat incurable skin ulcers and flesh eating infections [67].

Among the various topical uses of clay, for general detoxification I prefer clay baths which, while somewhat messy, are well worth the effort. Large amounts of clay are needed for baths, and the clay I use is designated as Microfine Volclay HPM-20 by American Colloid Company [71]. It is a fine-mesh high purity sodium bentonite clay which I purchase in 50 pound bags from Laguna Clay, a nationwide distributor [72]. To prepare the bath, while it is filling, hand distribute the clay on the surface almost as if you were sowing seeds, to avoid clumping as much as possible (some of which will happen anyhow). The more clay the better from a detox point of view, and the typical range is from 2 to 20 pounds at one time. The bath setting I use is a water temperature around 100 degrees F, and I stay in it for 20-30 minutes. The wet clay becomes very slippery, so care is required getting in and out of the tub. Draining the bathwater is straightforward, and only minimal cleanup is required. Municipal sewer systems apparently have no problem with the hydrated clay, but there is some concern that septic systems may eventually become clogged. I again refer you to Jason Eaton's site for some of the healing effects of clay baths, including Jason's personal story [67]. The frequency of clay bathing is a personal choice ranging from once per month to several times a week.

Humic/Fulvic Acids

These acids are a normal component of soil, and are known to bind with mercury and also to methylate it, potentially making it more toxic. However, regarding methylation, there is also evidence that the normal bacteria in our gut methylates mercury, so I do not regard this as a sufficiently important risk to disregard the use of these useful compounds [73] [74] [75]. A Hungarian company, Humet, has extracted a humic/fulvic acid compound they call HumiFulvate® from a peat bog in Hungary and have studied it as a heavy metal detoxifier [76]. The product is available in the U.S. as Metal Magnet™ by PhytoPharmica [77]. From my research on humic and fulvic acids, they appear to act as bioaccumulators, able to bind with heavy metals, and to let go of them easily, which is where the alkalinity protocol will come into play. One to two capsules per day during short-term detoxification is an average dose.

Spore-Forming Bacteria

Next, we come to the important topic of spore-formers. Their ability to stimulate the immune system, to generate unique antimicrobials that disseminate system wide, and to competitively exclude pathogens from taking up residence in the gut make them ideal agents to be used in a variety of detox protocols. Of the two spore-former species I discussed above, bacillus laterosporus has a history of controlling Candida overgrowth in even the most difficult of cases, and the developer of this spore-forming strain, Boyd O'Donnell, has obtained a patent covering its use as an antifungal (US Patent No. 5,455,028). Spore-formers adsorb minerals, so it is very important to use the mineral repletion protocols described. I stay on a maintenance dose of one per day to ensure I keep the gut flora under control. Undoubtedly, spore-formers also act as a fungicide and do kill off some Candida, but I have found the side effects to be minimal, such as occasional diarrhea.

Dolomite

Last on the list is dolomite. Dolomite is widely used in pollution control systems to adsorb heavy metals from flue gasses, polluted stream water and even lakes [78] [79]. In the case of lakes, an experiment has been proposed where large quantities of dolomite are added to increase the water pH in an attempt to reduce the methylation of mercury in the water. I do not know of any research on the use of dolomite in humans to remove or render harmless heavy metals, but it is quite persuasive from the wide scale use in industry that it has such an effect.

The Dirt Detox Protocol

For this protocol, for which a patent application has been filed, I have combined several natural substances. The goal is to determine if there is a synergistic detox effect in the combination that may make it more effective than the individual components. Perhaps it may be even more effective than the conventional detox protocols that are presently in use, particularly for removal of heavy metals.

The basic concept for this protocol is to combine clay, fulvic/humic acids, and spore-forming bacteria with alkalizing agents (including dolomite) that ensure the urine pH is neutral or alkaline. The rationale for this protocol is that each of the soil components individually is known to bind with metals in soil, and the strength of the soil-metal bond in each case is increased in an alkaline environment. What I am counting on is that the pH factor as applied in the human body will be the answer to the long-standing question for many detox protocols as to how to ensure that the detox agent does not let go of the toxic metal before it is excreted from the body.

The alkalizing agents can take the form of more fruit in the diet, dolomite, and/or supplements such as magnesium and potassium citrate. Here is an example of how I combine the individual components for detox purposes. Twice a day, upon arising and at bedtime, I take each of the following, all of which have been previously described: Pascalite clay (2 capsules), Immune Boost 77 (1 capsule), and Flora-Balance (1 capsule). In addition, during the day I take dolomite with water, as well as potassium citrate in sufficient quantity to ensure neutral to alkaline urine. Terramin clay tablets can be substituted for some or all of the Pascalite, Metal

Magnet can be substituted for one of the Immune Boost 77, and Lactobacillus Sporogenes can be substituted for one of the Flora-Balance. Sodium citrate or bicarbonate can also be used as alkalizing agents. Because the soil components are known to adsorb essential minerals as well as toxic ones, it is important to replenish minerals, some of which is accomplished by the dolomite. For a dosing schedule, I use this protocol for five days every two weeks, which allows for essential mineral replenishment during the off time.

Charcoal

Most people are familiar with the use of charcoal in emergency rooms for poison control, and in that regard, it works in a somewhat similar fashion as clay in that it adsorbs toxins from the body. Charcoal powder is somewhat messy to use because of its black sooty consistency, but it is widely available in capsule form under many brands. If clay is not available or not to your liking, activated charcoal caps, usually about 250 mg each, can be used instead, or they can be mixed together in powder form, which makes the charcoal somewhat less sooty. Like clay, charcoal has a long history of animal use. For example, after a lightning-caused forest fire, returning animals are known to chew on charred branches to get at the charcoal. The activation process used to make modern charcoal acts to increase the available surface sites for adsorption. Charcoal does not appear to have the high mineral content of clay, which might make it somewhat less attractive for use, and it will turn your stool black, quite harmlessly. Otherwise, it is an excellent detoxifying agent. There are several good sources for products and information [80].

Vitamins

I have found that, until a certain amount of detoxification has taken place, taking large doses of vitamins as supplements can be very counterproductive because they feed the bad guys. As an example, the yeast Candida loves many of the B-vitamins, and taking large doses can easily contribute to its overgrowth. Actually, some B vitamins are normally produced for us by the microflora in our intestines, such as vitamin B6 [81], but many of us have disturbed gut flora due to toxins, so supplements can be helpful. If we look to MA for guidance, we find that another major source of B-vitamins for PA would have been the liver of prey animals, probably eaten raw. Most liver lovers like to eat it fried, and the attendant high cooking temperatures may destroy much of the vitamin content. Another modern concern in eating liver is its potential toxicity.

Many people, including myself, have assumed that taking a B-vitamin supplement can provide us with the equivalent of what is missing from our food sources. It was not until I did some serious research into the nutritional advantages of liver that I discovered many animal studies that showed this is not necessarily true. Dating back to the 1950's, Benjamin Ershoff, a medical researcher, ran dozens of experiments with rats to determine the effects of various nutritive substances on the health of the animals when they are subjected to various toxins and other stressors. In several of these experiments he tested the use of B- vitamin supplements versus small amounts of raw desiccated (dried) liver added to the diets of the rats, who were then subjected to various stressors such as swimming, x-ray radiation, thyroid hormone disrupters and the like [82, 83]. In each instance, he found that the rats fed liver outperformed and out-survived those fed synthetic B- vitamins. His conclusion was there is something in liver that we are unaware of that provides benefits beyond just B-vitamin supplementation. I don't know of any studies directed to finding out what these substances might be. We do know that the liver is the major detoxification organ, and perhaps some of these detox agents remain in raw liver and provide a protective effect.

Armed with this information, I set about looking at the various raw liver supplements on the market to see if any would be a suitable addition to the diet. My criteria were that it had to be derived from organic grass-fed animals in a protected environment to avoid toxins, and it had to be processed using low-temperatures to avoid damaging the tissue components. A final criterion was that the supplement should include both the water-soluble and fat-soluble portions of the liver, because Ershoff found that the combination was an important factor in its efficacy. Several desiccated beef liver supplements are available that are made from protected Argentinean free-range grass fed beef, and they use low temperature processing. However, I could only find one that was not defatted. It is supplied by Now Foods as a powder or a tablet [84], and is the product I use as a basic B- vitamin supplement. (The appropriateness of additional B- vitamin supplementation is discussed below in the various detox sections.) I happen to like the taste of liver, so I chew five tablets at each meal, or put one teaspoon of the powder in my fruit tea. For those who do not like the taste, swallowing the tablets is the way to go. Because this supplement is really a food, you can munch on it during the day for an energy boost. There is a long history of bodybuilders downing fistfuls of liver tablets for stamina.

Before leaving the subject of B- vitamins, I want to single out what I (and others) consider the queen of this group, and that is vitamin B6. It is responsible for more enzyme reactions in the body than any of the other vitamins, and its proper assimilation is easily interfered with by a variety of toxins, including candida overgrowth. Studies have shown that consumption of sugars has the effect of depleting vitamin B6 in the body [85] [86]. The importance of vitamin B6 to so many of the body's processes, coupled with a higher sugar intake from modern cultivated fruits leads me to add a daily vitamin B6 supplement to my regimen as a precautionary factor. It is usually found in supplement form as pyridoxine HCl, which must be converted in the body to the active form, pyridoxal–5'-phosphate (P5P). Because some toxins, including Candida overgrowth, can interfere with this conversion, I take P5P directly. Further, because P5P is easily damaged by stomach acid, I take it in the form of a sublingual tablet, placed under the tongue to dissolve and directly enter the bloodstream. The one I use, at four tablets per day, is Coenzymated B-6, made by Source Naturals [87].

Vitamin C is in the news almost daily as either being a panacea for major illnesses or being demonized for one thing or another. First, we need some definitions. Vitamin C is found in plant and animal products. In animals, it appears to be in the form of pure ascorbic acid, and this is the form usually called Vitamin C. In plants, primarily fruits and leaves, it is also found in the form of ascorbic acid, but it is virtually always found along with a group of compounds called bioflavonoids which I will call the "flavonoid complex". In the animal world, all mammals except for a small group including primates, humans, guinea pigs, the red-vented bulbul (a fruit-eating bird), a species of trout, and the Indian fruit bat can make their own vitamin C. This group apparently lost the ability to do so, supposedly because ample amounts were provided in their diet.

Regarding vitamin C (ascorbic acid) supplementation, many of the products on the market are derived from corn, most of which is GMO (Genetically Modified Organism). Some corn-free products that are available are derived from cassava root (also called tapioca), or sago palm, all of which appear to be synthetically derived. I use corn-free Vitamin C 500 mg by Nature's Plus. I take one ascorbic acid cap with each meal.

Regarding Vitamin E, the very term is ill defined. It generally refers to alpha-tocopherol, which is found in nature only as part of a complex of tocopherols and tocotrienols. I try to avoid supplements that contain alpha-tocopherol as an isolated nutrient, since it is not found in nature that way and there is now some evidence that it may prove toxic in its isolated form. A better choice is a vitamin E complex supplement that contains several E components, including both tocopherols and tocotrienols. There are several such E-complexes on the market, and the starting material for many is red palm oil (see for example U.S. Patent 5,157,132). This oil is extracted from the fruit of the oil palm, which, lo and behold, is an Original Diet food. So instead of messing with the supplement products, one would ideally eat oil palm fruit, which is described as somewhat fibrous and oily. However, I am not aware of any readily available sources for the fruit. Instead, I suggest chugalugging some red palm oil (not palm kernel oil, which is derived from the nut), which is extracted from the fruit and which is readily available. Not only is it high in the E complex, it is also very high in the pro-vitamin A carotenoid complex, and in vitamin K.

Just as alpha-tocopherol is not found in nature as an isolate, beta-carotene is similarly not found that way, and I try to avoid any supplements that contain beta-carotene as an isolated ingredient. Some studies have shown that beta-carotene may be toxic in isolated form, particularly when Candida overgrowth may be present (see further discussion in fungal detox section). Red palm oil contains the carotenoid complex as found in nature, which includes alpha, beta, and other carotenoids yet to be defined. From my studies, red palm oil has the highest edible concentrations of Vitamin E and carotenoid complexes in the plant kingdom. Red palm oil is also high in vitamin K1, useful in controlling blood clotting, and as a raw material for enzyme processes in your body that helps keep calcium out of your arterial walls and bring it into your bones.

An interesting property of vitamins pro-A, E and K is that their absorption is increased significantly when consumed with fat, which is amply provided in the palm oil itself. I take one to three teaspoons of the oil per day, right off the spoon. The kind I look for is Organic Virgin Palm Oil, which is red in color, originates in Africa, and is not refined, deodorized, or bleached. One source is Tropical Traditions [88]. Red palm oil has been demonized as unhealthy because it is high in saturated fat, a red herring for heart disease [89]. For those who want to forgo taking red palm oil directly, a trio of supplements would be needed just to replace the pro-A, E and K components. Some suggestions would be CarotenAll by Jarrow [90], and *Super K* and *Gamma E Tocopherol/Tocotrienols*, both from Life Extension Foundation [91].

Vitamin D is another critical nutrient, and acts both as a vitamin and as a prohormone. The ideal natural source is from the UVB spectrum of ultraviolet light impinging on unprotected skin, and I feel confident that PA had no shortage of sunlight in the tropics. I already commented above on my theory regarding skin cancer, and I go into more depth on this subject in the lifestyle section. Modernly, unless you happen to live in a tropical or semi-tropical environment, it is quite difficult for people in Western societies to get sufficient sunlight year round to produce adequate vitamin-D, which has been found to be necessary for bone strength and it is a potent anti-cancer compound [92]. Alternatives to getting natural sunlight include an artificial UVB source using a UV bulb (discussed in the lifestyle section); obtaining vitamin-D from the diet (liver is a source); and obtaining vitamin-D from supplements. Serious research into Vitamin-D is just beginning, and there is much that remains unknown, including all of the various forms that make up what will undoubtedly become the "Vitamin-D complex" some time in the future. Because we don't know yet what we are doing in this area, the best course of action is to follow MA, and get it from UV.

I personally prefer a UVB lamp, but supplements are an alternative. Before taking any, I suggest getting a Vitamin-D blood test. The test is called 25(OH)D, or 25-hydroxyvitamin D, and the latest consensus seems to be that an optimum level is above 30 and below 60 ng/ml. Excessively low or high levels can be harmful. If the level is low, Vitamin-D3 supplements are available (avoid Vitamin-D2 since it is poorly absorbed and interferes with magnesium absorption). One source I have used is Biotics Research Bio-D-Mulsion (available in 400 IU and 2000IU drops). Getting to the right dose (say between 1200 and 8000 IU per day) requires experimentation and monitoring using the 25(OH)D test [93].

As is the case in so many of the tests designed to measure levels of various compounds in the body, the vitamin D test results have generated confusion. A study was conducted where the 25(OH)D test was run on a group of people in Honolulu who habitually obtained a great amount of sun exposure. It was found that 51% of the tested group had a test level below the 30 ng/ml lower cutoff, indicating vitamin D deficiency [94]. This leaves for speculation whether the test is unreliable or a large subset of the population does not properly produce vitamin D, even with significant UVB exposure. Until this discrepancy can be sorted out, I continue to prefer UVB exposure as the natural way to obtain vitamin D, on the basis that at least MA knows what she is doing.

Regarding the relationship between UV and melanoma, the most deadly form of skin cancer, there are about as many studies showing incidence increase with excessive sun exposure as those that show the opposite [95] [96]. Something I find puzzling in these studies is that it did not strike the researchers that those people who sunburn easily might also be those with a compromised defense system, making them more susceptible to cancer, independent of sun exposure. At lease empirically, it is well- known that, for example, deranged fatty acid synthesis (typical of eating the Standard American Diet (SAD) diet) can cause a person to be very susceptible to sunburning as opposed to tanning.

Minerals

The Magnesium Factor

The title of this section is borrowed from a very important book of the same name, *The Magnesium Factor*, by Mildred Seelig, MD [97]. As you will see, magnesium, of all of the essential minerals, is not only the most overlooked and most deficient, but in my opinion, is also the most critical to our health and very important in the various detox protocols. I will start with mineral supplementation in general, then move on to magnesium and finally to some of the support nutrients that work together to ensure an adequate supply of this critical nutrient.

Concerning minerals and Nature's Detox Plan, it would appear that PA derived certain of her/his minerals from two sources. The first is from food sources such as animal parts and fruit, and the second source is mineral water. Accordingly, I have divided mineral supplementation into two sections, one taken with food, and the other taken with water.

For food-based mineral supplementation, I take a multi-mineral to bolster what might be deficient in modern animal and fruit products. My preference is a supplement without copper (usually already elevated as a result of many toxins including Candida), and without iron (there is no shortage of iron in meat), and one where the minerals are bound to fruit acids. Examples of fruit-acid-derived compounds are citrates, fumarates, malates, and succinates. I also like a high magnesium/calcium ratio because of the importance of magnesium, discussed further below. There is no ideal mineral supplement, and they all contain human-made ingredients of one sort or another. I use *Citramin II* by Thorne Research [56], which is based on citric acid and is iron and copper free. I take three per day with meals.

For water-based mineral supplementation, the macrominerals calcium and magnesium appear in large quantities in natural mountain spring water. As you know from my discussion of water, I go to great lengths to ensure a high mineral content in drinking water. The water mineral content is dependent upon municipal water sources, which vary greatly, and the use of RO and distillation filters depletes water of these vital nutrients. One solution, mentioned above, is to supplement drinking water with small amounts of dolomite, which provide calcium and magnesium in the natural ratio of approximately 1.7 to 1. A protocol I have used is one dolomite tablet with water up to four times per day, for a maximum of four tablets.

While we are on the subject of dolomite, as mentioned earlier, the minerals that are present in mineral water are in the form of bicarbonates, while the minerals in dolomite are in the form of carbonates.

If we want to match exactly the bicarbonate form as a supplement, this can be done with some effort. Basically, mixing dolomite powder with carbonated water will do the trick. I have certainly experimented with this method, and have concluded that the carbonate form as found in dolomite not only has a long history of successful use, but works as well for me as the bicarbonate form. From a chemistry perspective, both the bicarbonate and carbonate mineral forms are expected to dissociate into chlorides in the body in the presence of stomach acid. However, I have found that orally taking chloride forms of these minerals does not produce the same positive results, so I intend to stick with dolomite.

Under "normal" circumstances, what I just described would appear to provide sufficient mineral supplementation, but we do not live under normal circumstances. Most of us live in a high chronic stress environment that has a major impact on depleting our body stores of magnesium, which I regard as the most important of all of the essential minerals. As you shall see from the following, I pay a great deal of attention to ensuring adequate levels of this mineral.

For this discussion of magnesium, I will be drawing upon the excellent research in Dr. Seelig's book [97], as well as the book *The Miracle of Magnesium* by Carolyn Dean, MD [98], and others. It is well recognized that those on the SAD diet have a deficient intake of magnesium from all of the processed foods being eaten. Further, as already mentioned, many of the seed- and nut-based foods in that diet contain natural mineral-binding toxins such as phytates and oxalates that block the uptake of magnesium as well as other minerals, so we may end up with a magnesium deficiency because of our modern lifestyle. It turns out that *stress* depletes magnesium in great quantities from our bodies, so that amounts that were sufficient for PA are not sufficient for us with our chronically stressful modern lifestyles.

Readers may take exception to the conclusion that PA did not lead a chronically stressful life, but the studies of modern hunter-gatherers show people who, for the most part, are happy, peaceful, and content with their lives. As previously mentioned, the fact that we do not make our own vitamin C tends toward the conclusion that, from an evolutionary perspective, our ancestor's lives were substantially less chronically stressful than our present lifestyle. I have no doubt that PA experienced times of acute (meaning short term) episodes of stress during hunting and predator evasion, but that is quite different from chronic stress that hangs around 24/7 in our modern environment.

Much has been written about the detrimental effects of chronic stress on our health, but there is little to pinpoint the relationship. Some believe that the increased levels of adrenaline and cortisol produced by the adrenal glands in response to stress contribute to illness, and then there is an entire "industry" devoted to the treatment of adrenal fatigue, which may well turn out to be the result of magnesium deficiency, usually in combination with a toxin overload. I can remember puzzling over the mind/body connection in relation to physical health for many years. How does stress make one sick? Well, Dr. Seelig maps it out very clearly. Everyday stressors that we take for granted, such as loud noises, reading the newspaper, listening to the news, politics, or even driving on the freeway cause our bodies to excrete large amounts of magnesium, which is needed for more than 300 critically important chemical reactions in our body. Physical stressors as simple as working in the heat or jogging use up or excrete large amounts of magnesium, as does exposure to toxins.

Magnesium deficiency can show up in many ways. Let's start with the one that first caught my attention: sudden death. I presume many of you can remember young, excellent athletes at the peak of health that suddenly drop dead when jogging. How about the patient that drops dead while on the treadmill in the doctor's office. Or the elderly gentleman who, in a fit of anger over some issue, grabs his chest and keels over. From my research, magnesium is the key to these disasters, and this is just the tip of the iceberg.

The above scenarios relate to the role of magnesium as a muscle relaxant, where it works in opposition to calcium, which causes muscles to contract. Some early signs of magnesium-related neuromuscular symptoms as a result of depletion include twitching, muscle cramps anywhere, including finger, toe, wrist, and back, heel and other bone pain, difficulty swallowing, headaches, tinnitus and hearing loss, spastic gut functions including reflux, and heart fibrillations. Further compounding the issue is the fact that magnesium interacts with other minerals, whereby a deficiency of magnesium can cause a deficiency of potassium [99], as well as zinc, and an over-abundance of calcium can interfere with magnesium absorption. Additionally, magnesium and vitamin B-6 assist each other in absorption, and the assimilation of this vitamin is, in turn, impaired by a variety of toxins.

A second major category of symptoms from magnesium depletion relates to its role in the production of energy. It is a critical factor in the production of ATP (adenosine triphosphate), which can be thought of as the body's batteries. Therefore, a deficiency of magnesium can result in serious fatigue and low exercise stamina. It is also thought by many to be a cause of Chronic Fatigue Syndrome. Now here is the Catch-22 with respect to fatigue. Many of the usual remedies to alleviate fatigue involve increasing the metabolism or energy state of the body, all of which require magnesium to do their job, further depleting the body's reserves and actually aggravating the fatigue.

Speaking of the body's reserves, much of the magnesium is found in the bones and muscles, so depletion can result in fragile bones and weak muscles. Depletion can also result in high cholesterol levels, and interference with essential fatty acid processing by the body. Magnesium deficiency is also implicated in kidney and gall stones, prostate problems, hyper-excitability, asthma, ulcers, depression, suicidal impulses, pituitary malfunction, and even body odor [10] [100] [101]. There are also studies that show magnesium supplementation halts the progression of polio if used early enough. By now, you probably get my drift that we are talking about a seriously important nutrient. A great deal of research on the effects of magnesium deficiency on the body can be found at several websites [7, 102]. Because it is involved in so many enzyme reactions in the body, the list of deficiency symptoms is very extensive.

I can personally tell you that if magnesium is depleted, many of the food supplements and detoxification remedies discussed here will not work and can produce adverse results. My analysis of this is that many of them require magnesium in particular to perform their functions, so they draw from an already depleted supply, thus increasing the depletion problem and leading to more symptoms. One example, discussed below in detail in the stress section, is the attempt to treat adrenal fatigue. It turns out that the typical remedies of hydrocortisone, DHEA, licorice, and thyroid hormone all deplete magnesium, and to some extent potassium, so it is quite important to achieve proper mineral levels before trying any of these remedies.

Magnesium replenishment is not so easy. The established approach for nutrient supplementation is to test for a deficiency and if there is one, to supplement to restore the level. For magnesium, there are challenges both to testing the body's level and to supplementation. For example, routine blood tests ordered by the majority of doctors do not test for magnesium. The standard chemistry panel only tests for three of the four body electrolytes (sodium, potassium, and calcium), leaving out magnesium, an incredibly important mineral. One reason is that a serum blood test for magnesium is virtually useless because magnesium is primarily stored in the cells. A more meaningful test would be a magnesium red blood cell test, which is a special lab order (meaning it costs more money), and even it is not extremely accurate [103]. A test that has been found to be more accurate in measuring all of the electrolytes is known as the EXATEST by Intracellular Diagnostics, Inc., and it may be covered by insurance [104]. This test uses cells scraped from the floor of the mouth to make the evaluation. Based on the test results, a supplementation program can begin.

Regarding magnesium supplementation, a problem with using oral supplements is a tendency toward creating diarrhea at the high doses that may be necessary to restore proper body levels. One method of finding the maximum tolerable oral dose is to increase it slowly until loose stools occur, then back off to a point where the stool is normal, referred to as the bowel tolerance point. Diarrhea should not be prolonged because it will flush most minerals out of the body, as well as cause dehydration.

Slow-release magnesium compounds have been developed in an effort to address the diarrhea problem, but the unknown with any timed-release or sustained–release product is how much is actually being absorbed in the gut. It is very much dependent upon the individual's gut environment, not exactly a controlled variable. One approach to oral magnesium supplementation is simply to ingest more magnesium carbonate, the form of magnesium found in dolomite. It is available as Magnesium Carbonate in 135 mg tablets from BodyBio [105].

There are many other choices for oral magnesium supplementation. Many of them combine the metal with either a fruit acid, such as citrates and malates, or an amino acid, such as glycine. A particularly serendipitous combination is magnesium and the amino acid taurine, which form magnesium taurate. Taurine actually exhibits some of the same properties as magnesium, and they complement each other in the body [106]. Further, as you will below, taurine can be of great use in alleviating the symptoms of Candida overgrowth. One brand of Magnesium Taurate capsules is by Cardiovascular Research/Ecological Formulas, widely available with 125 mg of magnesium per capsule. Another brand is Magnesium Taurate tablets by Douglas Labs, with 200 mg of magnesium per tablet [107].

I use either the carbonate or the taurate form in conjunction with the dolomite protocol. Daily magnesium dosages required to sustain normal body levels can vary widely from, say, 400 mg to 2 grams, and may be a function of one's toxin level (including chronic stress), among other things. For example, if you have high levels of lead, which accumulates in the bones, it may take larger amounts of magnesium to displace and replace the lead in the bone matrix.

Here are the oral magnesium supplement protocols that I have used in an effort to prevent diarrhea and assimilate large amounts of magnesium. I start with dolomite, and add additional magnesium as either magnesium carbonate or taurate or some of both. On an individual basis as part of the various detox protocols, and depending upon the toxin types and degree of toxicity being addressed, I would expect that daily doses of the various ingredients could typically range up to 4 dolomite tablets (containing 630 mg calcium and 350 mg magnesium) with 200-800 mg of additional magnesium. The dolomite tends toward constipation, and the magnesium has a laxative effect, so the objective is to balance the two to achieve normal stools and high magnesium intake. Taurine acts to stimulate the production of stomach acid, which assists in the assimilation of the dolomite.

Remarkably, even the above oral supplement protocol may not be sufficient to restore magnesium levels, or may take a long time to do so. One way to increase magnesium levels more quickly without causing diarrhea is to use a topical application. An established protocol is the use of magnesium sulphate crystals, known as Epsom salts, in bath water, which is quite soothing to some. Another protocol, and the one that I favor, is to wipe or spray on the skin a magnesium chloride solution - several such products are available. One that I use is Dr. Shealy's Biogenics Magnesium Lotion [108]. Apply an amount equivalent to about two teaspoons twice a day to random skin areas and either leave it on or wash it off after 20 minutes. You can also obtain from this same source magnesium chloride crystals for use in a foot or body bath. I believe the chloride portion of magnesium chloride will also assist in displacing toxic halides such as bromide from the body, which I discuss in more depth below.

I regard the topical application of magnesium as a very important adjunct protocol to aid in the restoration and maintenance of magnesium, and I plan to use it on a continuous basis. Dr. Shealy, a pioneer in the use of topically applied magnesium, estimates that it may take from 6 to 12 months to restore magnesium levels to normal using oral supplements [109]. For topical application, using the dosage listed above, he found that restoration occurred in 4 weeks. I apply the magnesium lotion twice daily, and I use a footbath several times per week with four ounces of the magnesium chloride crystals.

Still another approach to rapid magnesium replenishment is IV administration, as a slow drip of vitamins and minerals in what is known as a Myer's Cocktail [110], which usually includes magnesium sulphate. There are many variations of this cocktail, and the one I favor contains at least one gram of magnesium chloride. Ten drips may be sufficient to restore levels. Overdosing of magnesium is an unlikely occurrence unless a person has impaired kidney function, since excesses are readily excreted.

While all of the above magnesium replenishment protocols work well, I am experimenting with yet another one that I concocted and will discuss in the chronic stress section below. It is specifically designed to deliver magnesium to the pituitary and hypothalamus glands to kick-start the endocrine system.

As it turns out, saturated fat in the diet interferes with the absorption of oral magnesium supplements. The theory is that magnesium binds with the fat in the gut to form insoluble salts, unusable by the body. Looking at PA's diet, where much of the magnesium was likely supplied by mineral-rich water, it is likely that a portion of his/her intake of magnesium occurred between meals, away from fat intake. So I take some of my magnesium and other mineral supplements with my water away from meals.

In its role as a detoxifier, magnesium has been found to displace and replace lead from the bone matrix, and is also known to increase the excretion of aluminum and cadmium [111]. Magnesium may well prove to be an alternative to EDTA (ethylene diamine tetra-acetic acid), a lead chelator, in the removal of lead from the body [112]. (A chelator is a compound capable of forming an ionic bond with a metal.) There is also evidence that magnesium can be used prophylactically to inhibit lead and cadmium from depositing in the body [113] [114]. While there is not much in the way of research into the role of magnesium in detoxification, I believe it will be shown in the future to be enormously effective in dealing with many areas of toxin accumulation other than that of heavy metals. Of course, its ability to eliminate body odors of all sorts is another indication of its detox potential. Its uses in specific detox protocols will be discussed below.

Now, let's look at some of the cofactor nutrients that work with magnesium. Vitamin B6 is an important cofactor that aids in magnesium (and calcium) absorption in the body and is interfered with by many toxins, more reason to add it to the supplement list [115] [116]. Zinc is another mineral that appears to be depleted by many toxins, and it also requires sufficient body magnesium levels before it can be replenished. There is an interesting test, known as the Bryce-Smith zinc taste test (ZTT) [117], that is sometimes useful to gauge body zinc sufficiency, and here is how it works. You place about half a teaspoon of zinc sulphate solution in your mouth and swish it around for about 10 seconds. The objective is to experience a bitter taste somewhat immediately, indicating sufficient zinc, which is associated with the sense of taste. Delayed or no taste response is indicative of concomitantly lower zinc levels. Zinc sulphate solutions for use in this test are available from Biotics Research as Aqueous Zinc [118]. In the event of a deficiency, I have used zinc citrate and OptiZinc supplements (widely available).

The objective is to begin zinc supplementation and, about once per week, redo the taste test until the desired result is achieved; then reduce the supplementation to a maintenance dose. My personal experience has been that until magnesium levels are restored, it is impossible to pass this test, regardless of how much zinc is taken. I take 50 to 75 mg per day. Potassium supplementation is also usually required when magnesium levels have been depleted. My preference is to use potassium citrate (widely available), since it is also alkalizing. Dosing for potassium is discussed in the alkalinity section below, and is based on urine pH. Note that anyone with impaired kidney function or who is taking diuretics should consult their doctor before using potassium supplements. If more than 1000 mg is required to maintain alkalinity during detoxing, blood testing of potassium levels is suggested.

As you will see from my discussion in the lifestyle section below, I am not a fan of putting products on the skin that contain unnatural ingredients. However, there are some products with a low potential toxicity that can be used for a short period of time as an aid to restoring essential minerals and, for those, I make an exception. In the case of zinc, there are topical supplementation products available such as a zinc sulphate cream by Kirkman Labs [119].

While it would be great if we could normalize mineral levels before beginning detoxification, this may not be possible because of the effect of the toxins themselves. For example, mercury and other heavy metals along with Candida overgrowth can so derange mineral transport in the body that it is difficult to normalize magnesium, potassium, zinc and other essential minerals until the toxin load has been somewhat reduced. Therefore, the idea is to begin mineral repletion in parallel with detoxification.

Iodine

There is a very exciting story to be told about iodine, one of the body's essential minerals, and for me it illustrates how difficult it can be at times to tell whether a reaction to a compound is an allergic one or a die-off reaction resulting from some detoxification process. The conventional wisdom regarding iodine has been that its primary function is in the production of thyroid hormones, and with insufficient intake, goiter (an enlargement of the thyroid gland that resembles a swollen neck) will result. The RDA for iodine, an essential element, is 150 micrograms, which was chosen as the dose necessary to prevent goiter.

Iodine is one of the halogen family of minerals, including chlorine, fluorine, bromine, and astatine (which is a radioactive element). Doses of iodine that exceed the RDA have been thought to be toxic because of the symptoms that arise. These symptoms can include unstable thyroid activity, seemingly creating hypo- or hyperthyroid conditions, a variety of skin problems known as iododerma, and a cluster of other symptoms called iodism, including excess salivation, fever, acute runny nose, swelling and tenderness of the salivary glands and tear ducts, and canker sores. Some years ago, in experimenting with supplements naturally high in iodine, such as kelp, I experienced virtually all of these symptoms, declared myself allergic to iodine, and stayed away from it. That is, until I met up with those MDs whom I refer to as the three musketeers of iodine research: Guy Abraham [120], David Brownstein [121], and Jorge Flechas [122]. Over the last three years or so, they have joined together in an Iodine Project [123] devoted to researching the health aspects of iodine and how it really interacts with the body, the results of which have been startling. I will discuss some of this research in more detail in the section below entitled "The Halogen Problem." A lot of this research is still quite new, and much of the medical community is either unaware of it, or in their usual fashion, dismissing it.

At this point of the iodine discussion, I will highlight some of their findings, while referring the reader to an excellent book on the subject by Dr. Brownstein: *Iodine, Why You Need It, Why You Can't Live Without It* [124]. In the realm of detoxification, Abraham, Brownstein, and Flechas discovered that iodine acts to displace the other halogens (which are toxic in all but the smallest amounts) from iodine receptor sites in the body, restoring health. During this displacement activity, symptoms appeared that were believed to be allergic reactions to iodine, but actually were signs of toxic-halogen detoxification. In the realm of general health, they found that the thyroid gland was just one "user" of iodine in the body, and that in the female, the breasts and ovaries are also large users.

They developed a simple urine test to evaluate the body iodine status, and I suggest that everyone take this test, which can also be ordered from the Flechas website [125]. Out of their research also came an iodine supplement in the form of a tablet called Iodoral, and it is a convenient way to supplement if the test establishes a need. Both Iodoral and the test kit can be ordered from Vitamin Research Products [126]. They also discovered, based on both research and common sense, that the iodine RDA is set too low by a factor of somewhere between 100 and 300. Healthy Japanese routinely consume about 100 times our RDA, or about 15 milligrams of iodine per day.

As explained in Dr. Brownstein's book, the urine test will evaluate your present level of iodine sufficiency. Once a supplement regimen is in place, periodic tests can monitor your improvement. Virtually everyone tested so far (thousands of people) have shown iodine deficiency. Besides being a detoxification agent with respect to other halogens, iodine is also a powerful antibiotic and antiviral, and is probably the most popular choice of doctors and hospitals worldwide for wound disinfection in the form of povidone iodine products like Betadine®. Last, but certainly not least, iodine in the elevated doses mentioned above has been shown to eliminate cysts of all kinds, including breast fibro cysts and ovarian cysts. To me, anyone with a cyst problem anywhere on their body could benefit from iodine supplementation. In addition, ongoing research into iodine insufficiency and its impact on thyroid illnesses and cancers of all kinds is producing very positive results.

The type of iodine used for supplementation is extremely important. Human-made organic iodine compounds are, in general, highly toxic and should not be used. Also, avoid the drugstore tincture disinfectants, as many are toxic for internal use because they contain wood alcohol. For the last 100 years or so, doctors routinely used an inorganic solution called Lugol's solution, a liquid with one drop containing 6.25 mg of elemental iodine, comprising 5% iodine and 10% iodide as the potassium salt. The suggested daily intake for iodine supplementation was about 12.5-37.5 mg of elemental iodine (2-6 drops). Lugol's was widely available at this potency until very recently, when the DEA stepped in and decreased the potency of the OTC (Over The Counter) product sold in any quantity over one ounce, to less than half the original. There are several sources of Lugol's solution [127]. As I indicated earlier, it is best to be tested before using either Iodoral tablets or Lugol's solution as a supplement, and then use the dosages described in the Brownstein book.

For experimenters, while waiting for test results, you might have an interest in the topical iodine test. It involves painting some Lugol's on clean skin in, say, a 2-inch circle or square. It will stain the skin a typical orange color (it also stains clothes until it dries). Note the time of application, and peek at the spot every few hours. The objective is to see how long the stain remains visible. The rule of thumb is that if the stain disappears in less than 24 hours, you are iodine deficient. Repeated daily applications on different areas of the body has been known to extend the stain time, so it seems likely that transdermal absorption of some sort is taking place, with the body decreasing its rate of absorption as its iodine stores are replenished.

This is a very crude test because there are so many variables such as the evaporation rate of the liquid from the skin, and the absorption characteristics at different parts of the body, so don't expect highly consistent results. Once the stain stays for, say, 24 hours, the idea is to cut back the application, and just use the test occasionally, say once per week, to monitor level. Women who have applied the solution to the breast area have reported significant decreases in breast cysts. Various oral iodine dosing schedules can be found below for different applications. As a general precaution for anyone taking thyroid (or possibly other) hormone therapy, taking iodine supplements may require an adjustment of the dose of one or more of these hormones. Others and I have also found that large doses can radically affect thyroid test results until the thyroid reaches a normalized state, which may take some time. As an example, the thyroid hormone TSH may be elevated for as long as six months on this protocol. Note that for highly toxic people, even the skin test can provoke symptoms of a die-off reaction.

Other than for detoxification purposes, iodine is a great antiseptic, especially for topical applications. However, one annoying side effect of the topical use of iodine, other than for the skin test above, is that it *does* stain the skin, which, for some people, has limited its antiseptic applications because of cosmetic issues. To overcome this objection, I came up with a combination of iodine and clay (see side box entitled Clayodine™), which enables topical iodine to be used without staining. Moreover, the antibiotic, antifungal, and antiviral properties of iodine are now combined with the toxin adsorption characteristics of clay.

Note that this application is different from the de-colorized iodine preparations on the market, which are typically potassium iodide, not iodine, and they lack many of the antiseptic qualities of iodine itself. The Clayodine preparation is intended for antiseptic use, not detoxification use, where the preferred products are Iodoral tablets and Lugol's solution.

Clayodine™

I ran several experiments in an effort to remove the skin-staining effects of iodine without compromising its antiseptic properties. The result was a combination of two of my favorite detox compounds, iodine and clay. Some of the applications are poultices, bandages, toothpaste, mouthwash, gargle, soap, shampoo, a cosmetic base for troubled skin, and, of course, internal consumption. Here is how it works. For topical applications, first mix clay (e.g. Pascalite, Terramin, or Redmond) and water to form a mixture whose consistency fits the application (e.g. thick for a poultice, thin for a shampoo). Then mix the iodine (typically Lugol's Solution) with the hydrated clay to a maximum concentration, which is arrived at by experiment. The objective is to find the limit of iodine at which the combination does not stain the skin when used topically. This amount may be different for different clay compositions. For non-topical applications (see the lifestyle section for toothpaste), the iodine can be added to dry clay up to a maximum concentration where the iodine remains adsorbed in the clay. A patent application is pending.

Salt

If you read *The Original Diet*, you will find that PA's diet made available large quantities of salt from animal blood. Drinking blood is not convenient for me, so I supplement my diet with an unrefined ancient seabed salt. I avoid all refined salts such as common table salt and most other salts, even those labeled as "sea salt." In the unrefined category, there are those salts that are harvested from the ocean, and those that are harvested from ancient seabeds that have been buried for millions of years. The latter are my preference simply because of the currently contaminated state of our oceans, and the fact that we have yet to identify all of these contaminants, let alone measure them. In theory, ancient seabeds have been protected from modern pollution, and the odds are higher that they have avoided modern contaminants. The one I use is *RealSalt* from Redmond Incorporated in Utah [128]. There are some ancient seabed salts advertised from various other parts of the world, but I am skeptical of the quality control and test methods used.

Salt has the ability to cause the removal of toxins from the body in ways that we do not understand. Its uses in specific detox protocols will be discussed below. I love salt, use it to taste, and estimate I consume about 2 grams per day. Am I worried about high blood pressure? No. My resting blood pressure ranges from 90/50 to 110/60. An excellent book on the healthy aspects of salt, also showing that, for the most part, the increase in blood pressure from salt is a transient one, is *Salt: Your Way to Health* by David Brownstein [129].

Herbs

In addition to looking for clay, animals with gut problems also go searching for particular plants to cure themselves. Generally, these are bitter to the taste and contain what would normally be toxic compounds, not eaten for food. One objective is to use the plant toxins to kill or at least dislodge parasites from the gut, which is a major and recurring problem in the animal world. As you will see in the parasite discussion below, it is also a major but usually ignored problem for humans.

Fiber

Natural fiber, such as found in fruit, has been shown to have a detoxifying effect in at least some applications where the toxin binds with bile. Because the body recycles most of the bile during the normal digestive process, these toxins can remain in the body for a long time. Fiber can act as a bile-sequestering agent, binding up some of the bile, which is then excreted, as opposed to being recycled in the normal manner.

For detoxification purposes, particularly when the target is mold, it may be advantageous to increase the amount of fiber in diet by using a supplement. The easiest way to do that is to add fruit pectin, such as apple pectin [130]. There are many pectin supplements on the market, but many are made with the rind and other parts of the fruit that are not acceptable. One example of a product I have used is *Apple Pectin USP* by TwinLab at two capsules per meal [131]. Large amounts of fiber can also interfere with essential mineral absorption, so I see no reason to go overboard on quantity.

Chapter 6 - Specific Detox Problem Areas

In this section, it is my intention to discuss specific physical toxin problem areas prevalent in today's environment, along with some targeted detox protocols others and I have used with some success. In the following section, I will discuss emotional detoxification protocols.

The Incompatible Food Problem

In *The Wellness Project* and *The Original Diet*, I go to some length to define a diet that would likely have been the one eaten by PA for most of the 2.5 million year heritage of our ancestors. It has the lowest levels of natural toxins, which are those toxins placed by nature to discourage predators from eating certain of her plants. That diet can also be found in my book *The Original Diet*. The general food categories that make up the diet are listed below in Table 2. The basis for that diet is as follows: if we do not eat foods that are compatible with our evolutionary heritage, we may well be toxifying our body with each meal. For purposes of this book, I would suggest to those readers interested in embarking on a detox program to consider switching to such a diet at least for those days when detoxing. Some food and supplement schedules are provided in Appendix B.

The Chronic Stress Problem

You might wonder why stress is listed as a toxin problem area, but its effect on the body and on detoxification in general is so pervasive, it deserves star billing before discussing some of the other toxin protocols. In the magnesium factor section, I outlined the relationship between stress and magnesium depletion, and much of what I cover in this section is an extension of that relationship.

Table 2
The Original Diet

Here are the general food categories for the low natural toxin Original Diet:

- Animal protein and fat, including glands and other organs, from free-range hormone/antibiotic-free animals that eat their natural diet
- Non-Bitter Ripe Fruit - organically grown
- Soil: humic/fulvic acids and spore-forming bacteria
- Mineral-rich water with a high content of magnesium
- Natural supplements such as unrefined salt and glandulars to replace missing nutrients

When I refer to chronic stress, I mean any activity or event that stimulates the fight-or-flight impulse in the body for long periods of time. The range of precipitating events can be everything from loud noise to a life-threatening experience. Under stress, the adrenal glands in particular are responsible for generating large quantities of certain hormones including forms of adrenaline and cortisol. All of these activities act to deplete the body stores of magnesium, B-vitamins, and vitamin C. The amount of such depletion is affected by genetic heritage, acclimation to stress, and stress reduction activities. There are endless activities that have been featured as stress reducing, such as yoga, tai chi, meditation, prayer, and the like, and I will not go into details regarding these, other than to say that any activity that reduces stress is certainly advisable.

Anyone leading a high stress lifestyle may want to consider large doses of the B-vitamin group as well as vitamin C, and this is quite easy to accomplish, with the caveat that high doses of B vitamins may interfere with certain other detox protocols, as discussed below. One B-vitamin exception that bears mentioning is vitamin B-5 (pantothenic acid), and a biologically active form of it called pantethine. Neither appears to feed the bad guys in the gut, and instead support the growth of friendly bacteria. Pantethine, in particular, supports the production of cortisone and other hormones by the adrenal glands, improves lipid profiles, and is an important addition to several detox protocols. They are discussed in more detail below. Vitamin B6 is also depleted by stress, increasing its importance as a supplement [132].

On the subject of adrenal glands, one of the more serious effects on the body of chronic stress is what is referred to as "adrenal fatigue," where the ability of the adrenal glands to continue pouring out the elevated hormones necessary to support the high stress level eventually becomes compromised. The result is general fatigue as well as a compromised defense system. Many protocols have been developed in an attempt to correct these hormonal deficiencies, and I will review some of them in this section.

There are several tests for measuring the hormone output level of the adrenal gland, particularly the hormones cortisol and DHEA. A saliva test is quite popular, and a typical severe fatigue profile shows low levels of both hormones [133]. There are dozens of programs out there offering support protocols with a variety of glandular and other products that go on for pages. A protocol using a prescription drug that works for some people is known as the Jefferies protocol [134], where small physiological doses of hydrocortisone are taken orally during the day to supplement the amount produced by the adrenals. If the total daily dose is kept below the level produced by a normally functioning gland (about 30 mg per day), none of the nasty side effects of pharmacological doses of cortisone occur. When it works, it seems to restore levels somewhat to normal, and the person feels much better and apparently can stay on it for years, if necessary, without adverse effects. Then there are the prednisone tapers, which are proposed to combat fatigue, but they require close monitoring, are adrenal suppressive, and can be quite dangerous.

I first experimented with the Jefferies protocol years ago, with negative results. While my adrenal tests indicated low cortisol and DHEA levels, taking the small support doses of cortisone aggravated all of the adrenal fatigue symptoms. Consulting with several MDs using the Jefferies protocol, they confirmed that a significant fraction of those who have tried it do very poorly for unknown reasons. After some careful experimentation, I realized that increasing the levels of stress hormones requires the support of magnesium, and if there is a deficit, the replacement therapy will not work, and the initial symptoms will get worse. Bringing magnesium levels (and iodine levels) up to normal, along with heavy metal and toxic-halogen detoxing, may completely obviate the need for adrenal or thyroid hormone replacement therapy or, as a minimum, will enable the successful use of some of the hormone replacement strategies. Remarkably, Dr. Shealy has found that restoring body magnesium levels also restores DHEA levels [109], leading to the intriguing possibility of hormone replacement therapy being a natural function of magnesium replacement therapy. Since magnesium is so intimately involved with hormone activity, I wonder what the effect of magnesium normalization might have on hormone issues related to menopause.

One of my theories as to why many anti-fatigue remedies do not work properly is due to the depletion of magnesium, along with vitamins B-6 and B-5. Pantethine has been found to support the production of cortisol by the adrenal glands, making this an important supplement for stress related issues. A more thorough discussion of pantethine, outlining its other benefits, appears in the fungal detox section below. As part of my detox protocol, I take a 300 mg softgel of pantethine with each meal, available from Jarrow Formulas and others [90]. I also complement it with the conventional form of vitamin B-5, pantothenic acid (widely available), which I take with every meal at a dose of 500 mg. Neither of these supplements appears to interfere with any of the detox protocols. Virtually any supplement that increases the metabolic activity of the body will require magnesium, and those people with toxins such as heavy metals or candidiasis are generally deficient. Therefore, I also view the protocols described previously for topical magnesium and sublingual P5P replacement as an important part of any adrenal fatigue treatment protocol.

On the basis that magnesium deficiency may be a precipitating factor in fatigue in general, and thyroid and adrenal deficiency in particular as the result of excess chronic stress, I propose the following experiment. Both the adrenal and thyroid glands are controlled by the pituitary gland, located at the base of the brain at about the middle of the head. There is research showing that magnesium is necessary for proper function of the pituitary [10], leading to the speculation that providing magnesium somewhat directly to the pituitary might have a positive impact on fatigue. When surgery is to be performed on the pituitary, they usually operate by going through the nose, as a short path to the gland. My approach was to create a magnesium nasal spray that could be safely used, in the hope that the magnesium could be sufficiently absorbed through tissue to find its way to the pituitary gland somewhat directly. See the side box labeled Magnesium Nasal Spray for the formula.

Another major concern for those under chronic stress is the development of cardiovascular disease (CVD), and that concern itself can act as a stressor! There is little doubt that magnesium depletion as a result of chronic stress can lead to CVD by causing calcium deposits in the arteries as well as causing arterial and heart muscle spasms. Interestingly, Dr. Seelig has shown that magnesium acts to regulate cholesterol levels in much the same way as statin drugs, by acting on a coenzyme known as HMG-CoA, but with none of the drug side effects [135]. So for those concerned about cholesterol levels, be aware that normalizing magnesium levels may result in improvement in all portions of the lipid profile.

Magnesium Nasal Spray

The source of the magnesium is a solution of magnesium chloride such as Cardiovascular Research's Magnesium Solution 18%, widely available. For a container, I empty out and clean a commercially available bottle of nasal spray with a removable top, and fill it with filtered mineral water (free of chlorine and fluoride). I add 10 to 20 drops of the magnesium solution per ounce of water, and shake well. For those who want to add a preservative, add one drop of either Lugol's solution or grapefruit seed extract. Spray each nostril several times per day. If a burning sensation arises in the nostril, dilute the spray mixture. While salt-water nasal sprays, using sodium chloride, have enjoyed widespread use, in this experiment, magnesium chloride (and some magnesium acetate) is being substituted for the sodium chloride. I have been using the spray for a short time without any difficulties, and I do notice an energy boost.

The Heavy Metal Problem

The term *heavy metal* has many definitions in the field of health, so for the purpose of this chapter, I am going to narrow it down to a discussion of two particularly nasty and prevalent toxic metals in our environment and in our bodies: mercury and lead. Many other heavy metals are also no fun to have around in excess. They include cadmium, antimony, arsenic, aluminum, nickel, palladium, tin, platinum, bismuth, and others.

I will begin the discussion with mercury and wish to advise the reader that from my research and personal experiences, mercury toxicity is intimately bound with Candida overgrowth, covered in depth in the following section on fungal problems. Therefore, I suggest these two sections be read together so that the entire spectrum of this toxic combination can be fully appreciated.

Mercury is considered the most potent non-radioactive neurotoxin found in Nature. A neurotoxin is a compound that acts on nerve cells in a detrimental manner, either disabling or killing neurons and other portions of the nervous system. Examples of other natural neurotoxins are the venom of bees, spiders, scorpions, and snakes. Human-made neurotoxins are chemical in nature, and include nerve agents used in chemical warfare, which, ironically, were developed from research into insecticides, most of which are also neurotoxins. Neurotoxins have many harmful effects on the body, from simple tremors to loss of body functions to death, and virtually everything in-between.

What do you do when a caring dentist places a compound in your body a few inches from your brain, one half of which is the most potent neurotoxin in Nature, in an amount that will slowly leak out as a vapor to all parts of your body over your entire lifetime? Well, I used to say thank you, pay the bill, and make an appointment to have more installed later. What do you do when a caring pediatrician injects into the body of your child (or perhaps you in the form of a flu shot) a compound including this same neurotoxin? Well, I used to say thank you, pay the bill, and make an appointment to have more injected later.

These dental and medical practices eventually may be recorded in the annals of history as possibly some of the most tragic technology errors in the fields of dentistry and medicine (closely followed by root canals and fluoridation, but more on those later). To add to this story, except for the financial issues involved, none of this would have taken place. In the case of mercury amalgam fillings (no, they are not silver fillings), they were developed over a hundred years ago as a cheap replacement for gold alloy fillings that do not contain mercury. In the case of adding thimerosal, a mercury-containing preservative, to vaccines, the motivation was to make more cost-effective vaccine dispensing systems where multiple persons could be vaccinated from the same vial. If individual dose glass vials are used, no thimerosal is required.

I do not believe either of these practices has taken place with evil intent or in any manner intended to cause harm. The reason I say that is because those connected with the development and implementation of these blunders have also personally been the recipients of these same blunders. I have many friends in the medical and dental field, and the majority have mercury amalgam fillings in their own mouths, as well as in the mouths of their family members. They have all been vaccinated with thimerosal, as have their family members. With this as a prelude, I do not believe it is productive to belabor the mistakes of the past in any more detail. I strongly support all the grass-roots efforts around the country to promote legislation to stop the damage, but until then, there will be endless arguments and denials, fueled by conscience and the threat of lawsuits.

Our real work ahead as individuals is to find ways of removing mercury from our bodies, and seeing to it that no more is intentionally added. The major sources are amalgam fillings, vaccinations, and seafoods. As I mentioned above, there are many adults and children that can withstand large amounts of mercury without ill effects, and then there are the *others*. At least among vaccinated children, it is looking like the *others* are approaching 1 in 150, which is the current autism rate.

Before beginning any mercury detox program, it is important to support the body with additional nutrients that mercury either depletes or interferes with. The list of such support agents could (and does) fill a book [136], but I will highlight some that I have found to be particularly useful. Several more are discussed in the fungal section below. Because mercury interferes with the transport of minerals throughout the body, the additional mineral support previously described, particularly magnesium and zinc, is important, and I suggest the testing of mineral levels before detoxing.

Liver and high omega-3 eggs are good essential fatty acid support foods during detox. Regarding vitamins, for some, the gut is so deranged from heavy metals that oral vitamins are not well absorbed. One alternative is a sublingual (dissolved under the tongue) coenzymated B-complex, available from Source Naturals [87]. Note that this supplement comes in orange and peppermint flavors. According to the company, the peppermint flavor is free of wheat, gluten, and soy, while the orange flavor contains trace amounts of these in the flavoring. One per day should be enough. Remember that we want to minimize feeding the bad guys. Another approach to non-oral vitamin and mineral support is the IV administration of vitamins in a Myer's Cocktail [110], which is a favorite IV mix of vitamins and minerals mentioned earlier. I try to have a set of five of these twice a year, particularly to boost magnesium levels.

Many other support supplements have been suggested during heavy metal chelation to make the process more comfortable, particularly in the realm of fatigue. The HPA/T (hypothalamus, pituitary, and adrenal/thyroid) axis of the body is particularly vulnerable to heavy metals. The thyroid will receive a lot more attention in the halogen section below. Adrenal exhaustion is the usual suspect for fatigue as mentioned above, but I have found that this is not always the case. The HPA/T axis involves a variety of what are known as closed-loop control systems, an area in which I have had extensive experience in connection with spacecraft design. I do not know if the study of endocrinology includes courses in control system theory, but it certainly should. The bottom line is this: what appear, via test results, to be adrenal or thyroid problems may just as easily be hypothalamus or pituitary problems. However, since endocrinologists do not know how to control those glands, the adrenals, which can sometimes be supported with small doses of hydrocortisone [134], and the thyroid, which can sometimes be supported with thyroid hormone, get all the attention. Enter magnesium, again.

There is some evidence that magnesium is a key factor in the proper functioning of the pituitary gland [10], and I have personally found that restoring magnesium levels can have a positive effect on restoring hormone activity. For example, a long-term program of oral, topical and IV magnesium supplementation restored my low body temperature to normal, where adrenal and thyroid hormone replacement alone failed to do so. Where possible, my preference is to support the glands with *The Original Diet* and wait for the detox regimens to restore the glands to health. I will have more to say about the use of cortisone supplements in the fungal section below.

There is controversy over the use of vitamin B12 supplements, based on the concern that this substance might act to convert some mercury compounds to methylmercury, a particularly toxic mercury compound. There is some scattered research on the subject indicating that such conversion is possible [137], but I do not believe B12 supplementation would normally be required on *The Original Diet* because of its naturally high concentration in animal food. There is also evidence that humic and fulvic acids can methylate mercury. However, they are so important in correcting gut issues - insuring healthy bowel elimination, a major detox pathway - that I have no concerns about using these soil elements, particularly in conjunction with the alkalinity protocol. Remember that the bulk of stool is gut bacteria, so having the right kind in the colon can improve bowel excretion of toxins.

Regarding amalgams, from the work of Weston Price, and from Paleo skeletal evidence, if we did not live a life disconnected from our heritage there would be no need, barring accidents, to ever visit a dentist, much less have cavities filled.

Dental restoration amalgams are typically a combination of mercury, silver, copper, tin, and zinc, and a threshold question is whether you have or have had them. Many folks believe they can merely look in their mouths for metal color to make a determination, but that is not so. In many cases, tooth colored crowns have been placed directly over amalgam fillings, and the only way to know if that is the case is either to consult detailed and correct records from your dentist as to what work was performed, or to have the crowns pulled to look underneath. X-rays cannot tell because the metal crown material hides what is underneath. By the way, gold crowns are really alloys of many materials including gold, and porcelain crowns are usually porcelain fused to gold or another metal alloy. Nickel and other alloys are also used for dental materials. One problem with having many different metals in the mouth is that they set up galvanic reactions, forming miniature batteries, with saliva as the electrolyte. Perhaps you remember making a battery by putting a copper penny in one end of a lemon, and a zinc nickel in the other end. That is what happens in the mouth, causing currents and voltages that can disrupt the entire nervous system and lead to all kinds of symptoms, which just add to the already long list of mercury caused symptoms [138, 139]. So, for a definitive reading on your amalgams, you need either dental records, or possibly crown removal, not a fun prospect.

Before we temporarily leave a discussion of amalgams, there is an indirect way in which you could have been exposed to large amounts of mercury (and other toxins) from the dental industry even without having amalgams installed. The source of that exposure can be a friend or family member who works in a dental office or in a dental lab, and you spend a lot of time around that person. Unless they practice some sort of decontamination, it is quite likely that they will bring home clothing, shoes, and other personal materials loaded with mercury. A particular problem is mercury or other toxins on shoes, which are then brought into a home containing carpeting. The carpeting becomes contaminated, and babies and young children playing on the floor acquire the toxins.

Moving on to vaccinations, if you have recently had a flu shot, it most likely contained thimerosal, the mercury preservative. Going back in time to childhood shots or those needed for travel, the only way to tell if they contained thimerosal is by doctor's records, if they exist, which should have recorded lot numbers for each vaccine. These lot numbers permit tracing by the manufacturer to see if it was a mercury-dosed lot. There are online sources to check the history of various vaccines and their ingredients that may be useful [140]. Thimerosal-containing vaccinations have come under great scrutiny as a potential cause of autism, which has now reached epidemic proportions. It is not rocket science to imagine the damaging effects of injecting large amounts of mercury into a child, and I strongly support all of the organizations attempting finally to get mercury and other toxins out of vaccines. If you find it necessary to be vaccinated, perhaps it would be wise to insist on single dose vials, and even then, to ask to see the ingredient list.

Next, we move to seafoods and sea vegetables, all of which have been contaminated by humans. Even sea algae such as seaweed, kelp and the like are also contaminated. After all, the way fish accumulate mercury is from direct or indirect ingestion of sea algae, which have the unique ability to bioaccumulate toxins, including mercury. I do not eat anything from the oceans.

From the above, you can get an idea of your lifetime exposure to mercury. Does everyone exhibit symptoms of toxicity from mercury exposure? No, once again there are those who, through past mutations and/or evolutionary luck, possess the ability to be exposed to large amounts of mercury without ill effect. One guess as to why is that they have the natural ability to mobilize and excrete large amounts of mercury before it can cause damage. Are you one of them? One approach to answering this question is to see if you have any of the symptoms. However, the symptom list goes on for pages, and is undoubtedly not complete. I would have a tough time categorically ruling out mercury, at least as a contributor to the worsening of any symptom I could think of, so that is really no help.

Next is testing, but unfortunately there is no test for one's body burden of mercury, short of an autopsy! Blood tests for chronic mercury exposure are mostly useless because the mercury is swept from the bloodstream into cells everywhere shortly after exposure. However, there is a specialized blood test to detect if you are hypersensitive to mercury. It is called the Melisa® test, and it can check for hypersensitivities to a number of toxic metals, including such seemingly innocent ones as titanium and nickel [141]. It is very worthwhile if you have or are planning to have metal implants for whatever reason. If you test positive to mercury hypersensitivity, and your history includes mercury exposure, it ups the odds that it is ruining your day.

A urine mercury test without a provoking agent (a compound to push mercury out of the body via the kidneys) is also not very useful because without a shove, mercury is quite content to stay in your body for, say, 30 to 50 years. The downside of a urine challenge test with a provoking agent (a large single quantity of DMPS or DMSA, described below) is that it can cause the redistribution of large quantities of mercury throughout the body. Another type of urine test is starting to gain popularity, one that indirectly measures the effect that mercury has on porphyrins, organic compounds normally found in the body [142]. It is called the Urine Porphyrin Profile Analysis (UPPA), and several labs offer the test. Derangement of porphyrins has been correlated with mercury toxicity, and the tests have been particularly helpful in diagnosing autistic children poisoned by thimerosal [143].

A hair-minerals test may be useful, and certainly was for me. Unfortunately, many folks carrying a large burden of mercury are not very good at excreting it in their hair, and so get a false negative. Many autistic children fall into this category. Another indirect way to use a hair test for mercury is to measure the essential and other non-toxic elements in the hair, because mercury is well known to cause deranged essential mineral transport. You can order a test which measures both toxic and non-toxic minerals through Direct Labs [144], which has an arrangement with Doctors Data, a well-respected medical laboratory [145]. Andrew Cutler, a chemist and past mercury toxicity victim, has devised methods of interpreting hair essential mineral test results in an effort to determine if mercury toxicity is an issue, and has written a book on the subject [146].

While the neurotoxic properties of mercury can wreak havoc with one's personality (e.g. the Mad Hatter syndrome and Mozart's madness) [147], there are some other clues that can point to a mercury problem, not the least of which is persistent Candida overgrowth. As you will see from a discussion in the fungal section, it is very difficult to eradicate Candida when mercury is present, and in many instances, it is counterproductive to try to do so. Another clue to mercury or other heavy metal toxicity is that supplements and other remedies don't work the way they are supposed to, and may even aggravate the condition they are supposed to alleviate. Yet another clue is dry skin with or without bizarre skin outbreaks. A final but significant clue is a gut that just will not behave, switching from diarrhea to constipation and everything in between, at a moment's notice. Spore-forming bacteria and magnesium play a major role in alleviating some of these problems while mercury detox is underway.

My personal opinion is that, if a person has amalgams in their mouth and also has health problems, there is a likelihood they would not achieve optimum health without proper removal. This should be followed by a detoxification program to begin to eliminate the lifetime of mercury that has collected throughout their body, including in the brain.

The mercury detox problem is somewhat more complicated because having amalgams in place limits the detoxification protocols that can be safely undertaken. If you wish to keep your amalgams, and yet are interested in some detox protocols, here are the issues. Because you have a large reservoir of mercury from your teeth continuously leaking into your body, attempting major detoxification can quickly overload the body's ability to handle the potentially large amounts. One result is that mercury can end up redistributed throughout the body, making you much sicker and potentially making it much harder to remove the now scattered mercury, not a good idea at all.

There are a few things others have tried to minimize mercury release from amalgams, one of which is to avoid chewing gum, since tooth pressure increases mercury excretion. Minimizing the drinking of hot beverages may also be useful to decrease excretion. The only detox protocols I can think of using with amalgams in place are the natural ones such as sauna, fiber, clay, spore-formers, and fulvic/humic acids. The alkalinity technique is designed to work with these protocols to reduce the amount of redistributed mercury, but I am not aware of any testing to support my theory. In any case, the mineral supplementation protocols, particularly transdermal magnesium along with sublingual P5P, are very worthwhile to support the body.

If you decide you want to get your amalgams removed (I did), here are some suggestions. The first step is to find a dentist trained in amalgam removal, which begs the question of "trained by who"? There are many removal protocols out there, and frankly there is no perfect way to remove mercury. The best you can do is to minimize the amount of mercury inhaled and ingested during removal. Of course, the next issue is what to put in its place. Ironically, most of the replacement materials are also toxic, containing various plastic materials including the ubiquitous bisphenol-A (BPA) of bottled water fame. Trading one toxin for another is not a fun prospect, but the reality is any foreign material put in the body will generate some toxic reaction.

Your dentist needs to be fully trained in replacement materials, which hopefully are not themselves toxic! There are materials compatibility tests that can be run for both crown materials and bonding agents [148], but they are not foolproof. After much research and a few false starts, I decided on dentists trained by a pioneer in safe amalgam removal. His name is Hal Huggins, and he is a dentist who has personally suffered from mercury toxicity. As a typical pioneer, he ended up with arrows in his back and license revocation for daring to question the mainstream dental community. He offers a dentist referral service on his website [149], which is a good starting point. My dentist, David Villarreal, in Woodland Hills, California, was trained by Huggins and did excellent work for my wife and me. Another organization listing dentists claiming to be trained in amalgam removal as a specialty is IAOMT, International Academy of Oral Medicine and Toxicology [138], and they have a referral service. For thoroughness, I would further check out the potential candidates by running them through a grass roots organization called DAMS, Dental Amalgam Mercury Solutions [150], which collects data from patients reporting their experiences with various dentists.

Going hand-in-hand with amalgam removal are the issues of permanently damaged teeth, raising the prospects of root canals, implants, and bridges. I am not a fan of implants because that is reintroducing metal back into the mouth, permanently altering the jawbone, and possibly leading to infections and cavitations. If you still wish to follow this route, a Melisa test would be of use to see if you have an intolerance of materials such as titanium. I discuss the folly of root canals in the section below on bacterial problems, and I consider this procedure another major technology blunder that can lead to potentially serious health problems for some people. In my case, I had a tooth nerve-damaged during amalgam removal, and rather than risk a root canal, I had the tooth extracted, using a Huggins extraction protocol, and a permanent zirconia bridge put in its place.

Let's say you have decided on a dentist for amalgam removal, and have chosen a replacement material (I chose zirconium oxide). Before beginning the procedure, it would be a good idea to find a practitioner skilled in detoxification therapy so that after amalgam removal you are fully prepared to begin removal of the mercury stored in the rest of your body. Such a practitioner can also advise you on preparation for the amalgam removal procedure. Unfortunately, finding detoxification support is not so simple, as most dentists are not qualified in this area and there are as many mercury detox protocols as there are detox supplements on the market. I have studied many of them, and my findings are listed below. In this discussion, I am presuming the reader is already following *The Original Diet* or something similar, because anecdotal evidence has shown that animal fat and protein are important to support detoxification. After the discussion of the conventional detox protocols, I will bring in the Dirt Detox Protocol as a supplementary or possibly even alternative approach to dealing with the heavy metal problem.

The first category of conventional protocols I will be discussing concerns those compounds that can be truly described as chelating agents. While there is a wide range of chelating agents in nature, for purposes of this book, we will use the strict definition in which the toxic metal ion is bound to two or more atoms of the chelating agent. For mercury, a class of compounds known as dithiols meets this criterion, but they all leave a lot to be desired. I would like to reiterate at this point that it can be problematic to use these agents if you still have amalgams in your mouth, because of the redistribution problem.

DMPS (2,3-Dimercapto-1-propanesulfonic acid), also known as Dimaval, is a pharmaceutical agent developed in the Soviet Union fifty years ago and is widely used in Europe as a treatment for mercury intoxication. It is not approved by the FDA for such use, but it can be obtained from U.S. compounding pharmacies with a doctor's prescription. It binds to mercury, lead, cadmium and arsenic [130]. It also binds to some essential minerals including zinc, copper, and chromium, which can be replaced through supplementation. There is wide disagreement as to how DMPS should be administered – whether administering it by IV, oral, or transdermal means is best. Drs. Klinghardt and Gruenn, mentioned earlier, both have wide experience in this area. My personal chelation preference, described in the Cutler and other references [136, 146], and one that I have pursued for some time, is low-dose oral administration, taken every 8 hours for three days every two weeks, and then repeated. The dosing period is designed around the half-life of the chelator (also true for other chelators) in an attempt to keep an even amount in the body, minimizing the redistribution of un-excreted toxins. Starting doses can be as low as 5 milligrams, and increased slowly while monitoring detox reactions. I personally do not go above 30 milligrams per dose for any of the chelators. The idea is to stay comfortable during the process. I would suggest consulting with DAMS Intl. for referrals to practitioners in your area who are skilled in these protocols [150]. I also believe in keeping the urine alkaline while taking DMPS in the anticipation that alkalinity will greatly enhance its efficacy, and may also reduce adverse reactions.

Another chemical chelating agent is DMSA (Dimercaptosuccinic acid), also known as Captomer. It is available over the counter as an oral chelating agent, and my preference would be to take it about every 3 hours for three days every two weeks, and then it would be repeated. A safe starting dose would be 5 milligrams, which is not easy to achieve because the available potencies start at about 25 milligrams, so you must manually split doses. Others and I find DMSA produces more gut related symptoms than DMPS, particularly with respect to Candida overgrowth, and this is discussed further in the fungal section below. My comments regarding urine alkalinity also apply here.

The third chelating agent is ALA (alpha-lipoic acid), a compound appearing naturally in the body in small amounts, and found in organ meats. It is widely available as an antioxidant supplement, but, unlike DMPS and DMSA, it has the ability to cross the blood-brain barrier and theoretically chelate mercury out of the brain. My preference for ALA is to follow the same protocol as for DMSA, taking doses every 3 hours. It, too, is only available in large doses, and needs to be manually split up for a safe starting dose. If tolerated, it can be taken along with DMPS or DMSA. There are some studies that show ALA may interfere with the production of thyroid hormones [151] and aggravate hypoglycemia [152] and, and for some people it can only be tolerated after a significant amount of mercury has already been chelated from the body. My comments regarding urine alkalinity also apply here. Dr. Broda Barnes, one of the early pioneers in the use of natural thyroid hormone, identified hypothyroidism (as well as hypoadrenal and hypopituitary issues) as a major cause of hypoglycemia in his book *Hope for Hypoglycemia* [153]. So, it should come as no surprise that ALA's interference with thyroid hormone production would also raise issues of hypoglycemia. Personally, I have found that many of the adverse symptoms associated with the use of ALA as a mercury chelator can be avoided if thyroid and adrenal issues are addresses prior to use.

Another chelator, EDTA, bears mentioning, and historically has been used for lead chelation, although both DMPS and DMSA also chelate lead [154], but more slowly. EDTA has also been used both orally and in IV formulations to open partially blocked arteries in patients with cardiovascular problems. The way in which this is accomplished is not well understood, but EDTA has antifungal properties (so does aspirin) and this may be a factor [155]. There have also been some studies that show EDTA can combine with mercury in the body in a manner that increases toxicity [156]. It may have some uses for those who are mercury-free and have arterial occlusions. As mentioned above, magnesium may well be an alternative to EDTA in the removal of lead from the body and in the transport of calcium from the arteries to the bones, where it belongs.

There are many issues surrounding the above chelating agents, with little agreement in the detox community as to the way they should be used and the outcomes expected [130]. A major problem is that while the chelators may initially bond well to toxic metals, the bonds are not strong enough to prevent un-bonding of some of it on the way out of the body, thus redistributing the toxins in a sort of "musical chairs" scenario. It is quite common to have a worsening of symptoms while using these agents, and cycles of symptoms that disappear and reappear quite randomly. That is why I suggest having a coach available who is skilled in supporting you if you wish to go this route. What would be a breakthrough is a chelating agent where the bond strength is sufficient to lock up the toxin all the way out of the body. Until that agent becomes available, we are stuck with the above protocols. Having said that, and as part of an ongoing experiment, I am pursuing the approach that alkalinity may be one answer to redistribution. For those interested in keeping track of new developments in this area, DAMS is usually an excellent source of information.

I will refer to the next category of heavy metal detoxifying agents as bioaccumulators for want of a better term. This category includes certain algae from the sea. If we back up and look at the fish/mercury problem, it becomes apparent that the chain of events begins with small fish eating sea plankton and algae, which accumulate toxic metals as well as organic toxins such as pesticides. The big fish eat the small fish, and the accumulation cycle concludes with humans eating the toxic big fish. For this reason, I avoid naturally occurring sea algae such as seaweed, kelp and spirulina, as they may already be contaminated. However, some enterprising supplement makers have devised ways to grow algae, particularly chlorella, in a clean environment so you can buy it uncontaminated. The thought is that by eating algae, it will accumulate the toxins in your body and escort them out. Well, maybe.

Anecdotally, there are mixed reviews on the use of chlorella for mercury detoxification, and I can think of at least one reason why. Clearly, when fish eat contaminated sea algae, they become contaminated. Well, it is not rocket science to conclude that contaminated algae is quite willing to give up its toxins to its host, so one inference is that the algae-toxin bond is quite weak. This leads back to the problem of how much mercury-loaded chlorella in your body will get excreted as opposed to being redistributed. For those interested in trying it, a well-respected brand of chlorella is Yaeyama, sold under various labels. My gut won't tolerate it, so my body has made the choice for me. There is some anecdotal evidence that a lactating mother with a mouth full of amalgams can keep mercury out of her breast milk by taking chlorella supplements, which is a very good thing for the baby. What is unknown is where the mercury ultimately ends up in the mother's body.

I will refer to the next category of detox agents as mobilizers, which actually covers all detox agents to some extent. In this case, I am limiting the list to those agents that simply mobilize, but do not bond with or excrete toxins. The presumption is that they dislodge toxins from their present location, begging the question of what happens next. For example, cilantro, from the leaf and stem of the coriander plant, has been attributed with some detox characteristics, probably as a mobilizer [157], and there are many products on the market that contain chlorella and cilantro in various formulations. Cilantro (coriander) has antifungal properties, which may contribute to its effect in mobilizing mercury, as described in the fungal section. In the case of mobilizers, the questions are what takes the place of the dislocated toxin, which was presumably sitting on a receptor site normally reserved for some good guy, and where does the mobilized toxin end up? This is really a rhetorical question, because I really don't expect anyone to have the answers.

The minerals iodine and magnesium fall into the mobilizer category, but they are unique because they act as displacers and replacers. In other words, when they push a toxin out of its location, they (iodine and magnesium) are the ideal elements to replace that toxin in that location.

The last category includes adsorbers which, in the natural detox agent category, includes clay, charcoal, fulvic/humic acids, and spore-forming bacteria, as discussed above. There are also products on the market that use modified zeolites (chalks), and some sellers make outrageous claims for these products. From my vantage point, it is hard to beat the natural agents. It is generally believed that none of the adsorbers are systemic in action, being limited to operating in the gut. However, users of adsorbers for detoxification report symptom relief that would appear to require systemic detoxification. Therefore, I think it is premature to make any statements limiting their action, even if they themselves are physically limited to the gut.

While the above discussion has concentrated on the removal of mercury, the same protocols may be used for lead and cadmium. In particular, magnesium has been found to displace and replace lead from the bone matrix, and is known to also increase the excretion of cadmium and aluminum, so maintaining body stores of magnesium, as discussed above, is definitely part of the heavy metal detox protocol.

As you will see from the discussion of fungal problems below, it is my belief that mercury toxicity and Candida overgrowth are intimately related, and hence the protocols in that section are very relevant for use in conjunction with those presented here to deal with the combined problem.

In summary, to simplify this section of the book for the reader, here is what I suggest. Given what I know now, after years of experimenting and researching in this area, daily sauna is my number one choice for heavy metal detoxification, followed by daily magnesium supplementation. Next, on a schedule of five days every two weeks, are alkaline urine, clay, and the other soil elements of humic/fulvic acids and spore-formers, which form the Dirt Detox Protocol. I know of no studies that would contraindicate the use of these items for people that still have amalgam fillings in place, because none of these items are chelators that might pull mercury from fillings.

For those that want to take heavy metal detox to another level, an UPPA or hair mineral test is next on the list if you wish to quantify your level of toxification. Depending on test results and dental records, amalgam removal would be next, followed by oral chelation therapy on a schedule of three days every two weeks, where these three days are not the same days as used for the Dirt Detox protocol. Chelation would include DMPS in small doses, using the protocols I discussed above, and ALA, also in very small doses. I find that if I take ALA with DMPS, I can use the eight-hour dosing schedule for both. I presume DMPS acts to clean up any un-excreted mercury mobilized by the ALA. Appendix B summarizes these protocols in chart form.

Let's take a closer look at the Dirt Detox Protocol as it is applied to the removal of heavy metals such as mercury, lead and cadmium. As stated above, it is known that fulvic and humic acids adsorb heavy metals, particularly mercury, and the product Metal Magic is a commercial example of this type of detoxifying agent. From the previously cited references, it is also known that spore-forming bacteria (biomass) adsorb metals, including mercury, cadmium and lead, and clay also has a history of metal adsorption. A concern in the past with adsorbers has been the weak bond, raising the issue of whether the detox agents will let go of the metal on the way out, redistributing it.

My approach is to use alkalinity as the "glue" to hold the metals to the soil elements. As a way of testing the efficacy of this protocol, I am planning a program of self-experimentation, paying attention to redistribution as evidenced by the reappearance of previously resolved symptoms. Further, I will set up a schedule of urine-challenge testing, where, similar to the DMPS or DMSA challenge test, I collect urine after administering the protocol, to see if and to what extent heavy metals are being excreted in the urine. Humet, the company that provides the active ingredient in Metal Magic, has observed some excellent results for mercury excretion in urine testing, using just the humic/fulvic compound alone. The results have been reported by Doctor's Data lab, and they can be found in the research section of the Humet website [76]. I am hopeful that the combination of ingredients in the Dirt Detox protocol will show even better results, and that this method may end up as a replacement for some of the conventional detox methods.

I want to emphasize the use of activated charcoal to quickly deal with acute detox symptoms, should they be experienced with any of the protocols. Charcoal's huge surface area makes it the ideal choice when you are suddenly hit with the typical detox symptoms of head, neck and shoulder pain. After much experimentation, I have found that, in my case, this is referred pain from the gut, and charcoal caps (10-15 at one time) can mop it up fast. Remember that doses of charcoal for routine poison control can range from 20-100 grams (equivalent to about 80-400 capsules!) Another fast-acting remedy for some detox symptoms is to add alkaline foods and supplements, as discussed above.

There are a few online support groups that discuss some of the various heavy metal detox protocols covered here, other than the Dirt Detox method. Look for Yahoo groups with the word *chelation* in the title. You will see as we discuss other toxin issues (even including the subject of indoor lighting) that mercury will continue to rear its ugly head. Which bring us to the fungal problem.

The Fungal Problem

A discussion of body fungal problems will usually center around Candida. Drs. Truss, Crook, and Trowbridge have been instrumental in uncovering the role that overgrowth of Candida and related yeasts (candidiasis) in the gut and elsewhere can play in causing illness. It is well established that taking large and/or frequent doses of antibiotics can predispose one to this condition, and often probiotics are prescribed in an attempt to prevent the problem. The theory is that the antibiotics reduce the bacterial population in the gut, allowing for fungal overgrowth. Well, that may be the start of the fungal problem, but it certainly is not the entire picture for many people.

There are many natural treatments for Candida overgrowth, and since I have had a very long relationship with this issue, I have probably experimented with most of them. They included oregano in all forms, olive leaf extract, grapefruit seed extract, digestive enzymes, pre- and probiotics, caprylic acid, undecenoic acid, tea tree oil, fiber, garlic, pau d'arco, artemesia, silver, other yeast products, EFAs, vitamin C, B vitamins, and others I can no longer remember. In the prescription category, I have experimented with nystatin, ketoconazole, itraconazole, fluconazole, amphotericin B, terbinafine, and clotrimazole, among others. Of course, I followed the various anti-Candida diets very closely over the years, as reported earlier. They all worked in their own way to alleviate symptoms, which were mostly gut and skin problems for me. However, for some reason, I could never really get rid of it completely. Re-enter mercury.

Candida is a genus of yeasts, and the *albicans* variety appears to be the most significant. It is found in our gut, skin, and mucus membranes and is very much a part of our natural environment. There are other Candida varieties such as *tropicalis* and *parapsilosis* that also hang around in our intestines. In fact, just as in the case of our gut bacteria, we are mostly clueless as to identifying the number and characteristics of all of the fungi in our intestines. There may be hundreds or thousands of varieties, and to complicate matters, they can easily change configurations from docile yeast to predatory fungi that can burrow through the intestinal wall and cause systemic infection. Studies of root-canalled teeth and cavitation sites (voids in the jawbone under teeth) show large concentrations of fungi, and a test discussed in the following section can detect them. One reason I do not like to see plastics used as dental restoration materials or even for orthodontics is that they apparently act as ideal surfaces on which Candida can form biofilms that are very hard to eradicate [158].

Mercury is an antifungal, which is one reason why thimerosal is used in vaccines. So at first blush, having a lifetime supply of it in our teeth and cells would sound like a good thing. We know, however, that prolonged use of a single type of antifungal can lead to the development of yeast that has become resistant to that antifungal. Could it be that the constant presence of mercury from amalgams, vaccinations, and fish can spawn mercury and antifungal-resistant yeast? You bet, but it only gets worse. For reasons nobody has yet figured out, yeast loves heavy metals, including mercury, and is happy to form compounds with them. Yeast has actually been used commercially to mop up heavy metal spills, and in mining applications to assist in extraction of metals. The upshot of all this is the creation of yeast that is resistant to most of the natural and pharmaceutical antifungals, as well as yeast that has bonded with mercury in our bodies [159] [160, 161].

There are many theories regarding the implications of the above information. One theory is that the body, in order to protect itself from mercury toxicity, will preferentially support the overgrowth of yeast so that mercury will bond with it, taking it out of circulation [162]. Ironically, one could thus look at yeast as a detox agent, which somehow bonds to heavy metals. However, unlike real detox agents, which escort toxins out of the body, the yeast/metal combination is quite happy to stay put.

Another theory supporting the yeast/mercury relationship is the following. Neutrophils are a form of white blood cell produced by the immune system to fight invading organisms, and they are a first-line defense against fungi such as Candida [163]. Unfortunately, mercury disables neutrophils, severely limiting their ability to control fungal overgrowth [164] [165], and as a result the body is unable to keep Candida in check, permitting a large amount of mercury-bonded Candida to reside in the gut and perhaps elsewhere in the body. Now, let's say you decide you have Candida overgrowth, and start taking antifungals to get rid of it. To the extent the antifungals are successful, you may inadvertently be releasing large amounts of mercury from the damaged yeast cells, and this mercury can now redistribute, potentially causing more damage than the Candida overgrowth.

In light of the above, others and I believe that wholesale antifungal therapy may be counterproductive for those who are mercury toxic, and a more realistic approach is to tolerate, to the extent you are comfortable, Candida overgrowth symptoms while at the same time detoxing the mercury. There are all sorts of tests available that claim to detect fungal overgrowth, including stool and saliva tests. I have found them to be less than reliable, with many false negatives. Another approach that has been proposed is to take an antifungal, such as nystatin, and see what happens. Supposedly, if you get an adverse reaction, you can assume it is the result of a yeast die-off reaction. Conversely, if you do not get a reaction, you supposedly do not have a yeast problem. While it is not a bad idea to try this test, it does not always work, because at most it proves that you no longer have yeast that is sensitive to that antifungal. As stated above, the mercury-Candida connection produces antifungal-resistant strains that do not die when you take some antifungals, so the lack of a reaction may not be a reliable indication of anything other than that the antifungal you are using does not work.

The detox community has found it most puzzling that the symptom list for Candida overgrowth is virtually identical to the symptom list for mercury toxicity. I am going to go out on a limb here, based on years of self-experimentation and research, and make the following statement. If you are mercury toxic, you will have a persistent yeast overgrowth problem, and conversely, if you have a persistent yeast overgrowth problem, you are mercury toxic – period. In fact, the two conditions are intimately related, which is why the symptom list is virtually the same. This really is not rocket science, and what follows is some additional research that has led me to make this conclusion.

Conventional wisdom has concluded that extensive use of antibiotics is a sufficient cause for a Candida overgrowth problem that continues even after the discontinuance of the antibiotic. However, not everyone that takes antibiotics ends up with fungal overgrowth, and many tests have been run on non-immunocompromised rats that show that the gut is quite capable of re-colonizing to normal after antibiotics have been stopped [166]. I believe it is mercury (and/or another heavy metal) overload, which works in combination with antibiotic or hormone use, (either of which itself can become a necessary cause of chronic Candida overgrowth), whereby the combination provides the sufficiency to sustain Candida overgrowth after antibiotics have been stopped. In the autism treatment community, it has become well established that kids with autism respond well to both antifungal therapy as well as mercury chelation therapy, again showing another strong link between the two conditions [167].

Some believe that Candida is limited to the gut and therefore could not cause systemic illness. Candida does not have to leave the gut to produce systemic illness. It produces dozens of toxins that can easily travel throughout the body to do damage. One of these toxins is acetaldehyde, described more fully below. It is also well known that Candida populates virtually all of the mucus membranes of the body, including the vagina and the sinuses. Recent studies have shown that most nasal, sinus and ear infections are really fungal in origin, and using antibiotics or cortisone-based medicines will seriously aggravate the condition [168].

Another parallel between Candida and mercury includes treatments that involve decreasing the amount of copper in the body. Most mercury-detox protocols include attempts to decrease copper, which also happens to be the same protocol for Candida control. It turns out that not only is Candida tolerant of high copper concentrations, copper also increases its virulence [169, 170]. It is also interesting that nystatin, a soil-based antifungal, is known to remove copper, and this may be part of its action against Candida [171]. Molybdenum is another link between mercury and Candida. This metal is often prescribed in mercury-detox protocols, and yet it is also quite important in supporting the enzymes used to render harmless acetaldehyde, a toxic byproduct of Candida. Thiamine (vitamin B-1) is yet another link. It is used as a supplement with some success in treating autistic children, and it is also found to be depleted by acetaldehyde in Candida overgrowth, probably as a result of magnesium deficiency (thiamine requires magnesium to function properly). Lastly, the detrimental and long lasting effect of mercury on neutrophils, a first line body defense against fungal overgrowth [165], seals the deal for me – we are really talking about what probably should be called the "Mercury-Yeast Spectrum Disorder™," so in keeping with "we name it we tame it," I hereby anoint this nasty disorder as MYSD.

Some additional discussion is warranted on the role of acetaldehyde in the Candida overgrowth matrix of symptoms, because I believe it plays such a large role. In *The Original Diet*, I described how fruit fallen from a tree can ferment in the presence of yeast, yielding a high alcohol (ethanol) content. When the sugars in carbohydrates are exposed to Candida in the human gut, the same thing happens, and ethanol is produced. It is then broken down into carbon dioxide and water in the same way that alcohol from an alcoholic beverage is processed by the body. During this process, which takes place in the liver and other organs such as the brain and kidneys, a potent neurotoxin is produced called acetaldehyde (AH). From my research, this toxin is the culprit behind many of the symptoms resulting from the mercury-yeast spectrum disorder, which, by the way, also shares many of the symptoms of the autism spectrum disorder, as well as many of the symptoms of chronic alcoholism! Yes, alcoholism. Because of the propensity for yeast to produce alcohol, it occurred to me (and others) that an overgrowth might be akin to having an alcohol still in the gut that is pumping it into our system 24/7. The amounts generated may be too low to be easily measured in the bloodstream, yet its persistence can have a severe impact on health.

I am now going to discuss AH in some depth, based on the combination of a chain of observations that look like the following. There is a mercury-yeast-spectrum-disorder, and it causes chronic alcohol production in the gut, leading to the continuous formation of acetaldehyde (AH), which may well be the cause of or a contributing factor for many of the symptoms related to this disorder. I will also discuss supplements that have been shown to offset the damage caused by AH and ethanol.

Dr. Truss, previously mentioned as a leader in yeast disorder research, came to this conclusion more than 25 years ago: there is a strong relationship between Candida overgrowth (candidiasis) and the symptoms of chronic alcohol poisoning. Much of the following information is derived from his important research paper entitled *Metabolic Abnormalities in Patients with Chronic Candidiasis – The Acetaldehyde Hypothesis* [172]. Dr, Truss, in turn, relied upon experts in the field of alcoholism treatment, including Dr. Charles Lieber, whose study entitled *Alcohol: Its Metabolism and Interaction With Nutrients* also forms a part of my discussion [173].

While most of the research that has been conducted regarding the adverse effects of AH is primarily directed toward the treatment of alcoholism, it turns out that much the same damage takes place in the mercury-yeast disorder. AH causes brain damage by interfering with the oxygen-carrying capability of red blood cells, and causes nerve-cell damage in a manner similar to that in Alzheimer's disease. AH induces magnesium deficiency, thiamine (vitamin B1) deficiency, niacin (vitamin B3) deficiency, coenzyme A (derived in part from vitamin B5) deficiency, and P5P (another reason for vitamin B6 supplementation) deficiency. It also interferes with the body's ability to use delta-6 desaturase to convert essential omega-6 fatty acids to GLA (gamma-linolenic acid), an important fatty acid for mood regulation and to control inflammation. AH binds to sulfhydryl groups, which are the very groups relied upon by the mercury and lead chelating agents referred to above, hence interfering with their detox action. On the other hand, this sulfhydryl binding also takes AH out of action, reducing its toxicity [174]. AH also bind to amines, the results of which are far reaching, including: abnormalities in porphyrin metabolism (which also happens with mercury toxicity and which lead to the UPPA test, as discussed in the previous section).

AH causes glutathione depletion (leading to free-radical damage), interference with liver metabolism of toxins, and derangement of amino acids in the body. AH also interferes with fatty acids, whereby most omega-3 fatty acid levels are depressed. It also uniquely increases the fluidity of membranes lining the gut wall, leading me to speculate that AH is a major cause of the "leaky gut syndrome" where toxins can pass through the intestinal membrane into the bloodstream. AH also produces opiates that cause cravings for things such as sugar and alcohol, which feed the cycle of further AH production [175].

I could go on for many more pages reciting the damage caused by AH and the uncanny similarity to Candida overgrowth and mercury toxicity symptoms, but I will focus on two areas in particular than can have far reaching effects on health, and for which certain supplement therapies has proven successful. The first has to do with the effect of AH on the membranes of the red blood cells. Although as stated above, the fluidity of gut wall membranes is increased, in the case of red blood cells, AH stiffens their membranes. This rigidity interferes with the ability of the blood cells to pass through many of the small capillaries in the body, and disrupts the ability of nutrients to enter the blood cells. The result of these disruptions can range from mineral transport abnormalities (this also happens with mercury toxicity), energy disruption, neurological symptoms, and nutrient and oxygen deprivation. Mitral valve prolapse, carpal tunnel syndrome, non-responsiveness to hormones, and imbalances of the autonomic nervous system are just a few of the problems that may be caused by the membrane stiffness effects of AH.

An unusual supplement has been used to overcome the effects of this membrane stiffness, and it is a particular form of phosphatidylcholine (PC) known as polyenylphosphatidylcholine (PPC). These are long words for fat-soluble molecules that are a natural part of cell membranes in the body, depleted by AH. From my research, there is only one source of PPC in the US. It is made and sold under the name PhosChol by Nutrasal [176], is also sold under the name PPC by Source Naturals, and is sold under the name Hepatopro by Life Extension Foundation [91]. It is derived from soy, not one of my favorite foods, but in this instance, the product appears to be devoid of the proteins and phytosterols that contribute to soy toxicity, so I use it as a detoxification supplement while dealing with MYSD. I take three gelcaps daily (900 mg each), one with each meal.

Liver toxicity is the second major area of health disruption caused by ethanol and AH. It is probably no surprise to anyone that chronic levels of alcohol and its metabolites delivered to the liver for detoxification can result in the classic symptoms of alcoholic liver disease. The supplement of choice in dealing with this issue is S-adenosylmethionine (SAMe), a coenzyme used to support the methylation pathways in the liver. It is sold under a variety of brands such as Source Naturals, and I take 200 to 400 mg twice a day, away from meals. There is also research to show that the amino acid taurine works in conjunction with magnesium, and protects the liver of rats from ethanol damage [177] [178]. It also acts to support neutrophils, the body's defense against Candida [179]. As you recall, one of the suggested oral magnesium supplements is magnesium taurate, which contains a substantial amount of taurine. Note that vitamin B6 also acts to support neutrophils [180].

I mentioned a unique form of vitamin B-5, pantethine, in the stress section above for its ability to support the adrenal glands. It also has been found to lower the blood levels of AH, apparently by increasing the activity of aldehyde dehydrogenase, an enzyme that breaks down AH to acetic acid [181]. Additionally, pantethine appears to have the unique characteristic of not supporting the growth of yeasts, yet it strongly supports the growth of healthy gut bacteria [182]. Add to this the fact that pantethine improves the lipid profile (in ways that are not understood), and you end up with an important supplement for both the fungal and stress detox areas.

There are additional supplement protocols designed to deal with AH by either binding with it or hastening its conversion to acetic acid by the liver. I have experimented at length with many of these and found that they either do not produce any meaningful results, or aggravate the yeast overgrowth. One set of examples is the taking of large doses of vitamins in an attempt to replace those lost due to Candida overgrowth. This can be quite counterproductive because Candida thrives on vitamins, particularly the B vitamins, including biotin, thiamine, B-3 and B-6 [183]. The B vitamin protocols I mentioned earlier, particularly the coenzymated sublingual versions of B-complex and B-6 appear to be a good compromise.

A vitamin-A supplement (unfortunately synthetic) may also be useful because it is depleted by ethanol, and one source is Bio-Ae-Mulsion from Biotics Research. I have used a daily dose of 4000 IU. It is my belief that vitamin A supplements should always be taken with vitamin D3 supplements to prevent toxicity, because they are almost always found together in nature in about a 10:1 ratio (in units of IU), such as in natural cod liver oil. As indicated earlier, I take 4000 IU of vitamin A, and I make sure I take at least 400 IU of synthetic vitamin D3. Additional information regarding the interactions between vitamins A and D can be found on the Weston Price Foundation website [184].

A caution is in order with respect to synthetic vitamin A and beta-carotene supplementation in the presence of ethanol. Lieber has found that ethanol both depletes vitamin A and potentiates its repletion, leaving a rather narrow window for supplementation, since excessive vitamin A can produce liver toxicity. I limit my supplementation to 4000 IU and feel comfortable that adding vitamin D resolves the toxicity issue.

The interaction between ethanol and beta-carotene is quite unusual. As I mentioned earlier, I do not take beta-carotene as an isolated nutrient, but always as part of a carotenoid complex. Well, studies have found that when beta-carotene was taken in combination with ethanol, it increased liver toxicity as compared to ethanol alone. I know of no studies related to the use of the entire carotenoid complex, such as found in red palm oil, but I feel comfortable that sticking with MA's formula will avoid adverse effects.

Yet another compound that has been found to protect the liver from the toxic effects of alcohol, and that is the amino acid glycine, found in large quantities in gelatin. It can provide long-term liver recovery and protection [185] [186].

Some in the Candida-supplement world believe that taking additional biotin will prevent the Candida yeast from converting to its invasive form, but that has been shown not to be true [187]. What keeps Candida happy in the gut is glucose. If it is starved of glucose, conversion to an invasive form is likely to take place, where it can burrow through the intestinal wall and become systemic. Now, let's move on to controlling this beast.

As I indicated above, trying to wipe out Candida overgrowth while you still have a significant body-burden of mercury may be counterproductive. Further, the body's defense system remains crippled by mercury, so that it is unable to control Candida regrowth. However, there is a program that I have used to control Candida overgrowth symptoms and some of the damage it causes. My approach is to minimize killing the fungus outright, all while continuing to reduce my mercury body burden using the protocols described above in the heavy metal section. A first approach is not to overfeed it, and I have found *The Original Diet* to be quite helpful in controlling Candida, even though fresh fruit is part of the diet. From my experience, the major Candida culprits related to fruit are dried fruit and fruit juices, both high in sugars and not part of *The Original Diet.*

Second, I try to support the immune system naturally by taking a supplement designed to do so. The one I use is called ProBoost by Genicel [188], which is a sublingual powder that contains a protein normally provided by the thymus gland, and which supports the entire immune system in a totally natural manner. There is substantial research on their website showing the efficacy of the product in relation to the immune system, as well as having a suppressive effect on Candida overgrowth[189]. I take one packet of the powder daily, but up to three per day can be taken if needed to help suppress infection. I consider this supplement of such importance in this modern world of infectious toxins that I have incorporated it as a part of my regular diet. Finally, a supplement based on the amino acid cysteine, N-Acetyl-cysteine (NAC) has been shown to reduce the damage caused by AH and to stimulate the activity of neutrophils [190] [191] [192, 193] [194]. NAC is a sulfur compound which can weakly bond to mercury and drag it around, so some mercury toxic people do not tolerate it. I have not found any problems using it along with the alkalinity protocol. There are many brands available, and I take one per meal of the 500 mg Jarrow Formulas brand N-A-C during detox [90].

While we are on the topic of sulfur compounds and Candida, there are conflicting data in the research community as to whether sulfur-containing compounds promote or deter Candida overgrowth. Sulfur is the third most abundant mineral in our body and is a component of every cell. In its elemental form, sulfur is a potent antifungal, and has been used as such for millennia. Of course, all of the mercury chelating agents are sulfur-containing compounds, as are SAMe, NAC, and an enormous number of foods. It is unclear from the research as to which sulfur compounds might feed Candida growth in the human intestine, if any. From my point of view, I feel comfortable taking these supplements in conjunction with the overall Candida control protocols outlined in this section.

Bad things happen when you mix Candida (and other yeasts) with cortisone – yeasts really grow out of control. The theory is that cortisone, a hormone, suppresses the immune system, allowing free reign for fungal overgrowth, as demonstrated by several research studies [195] [196] [197]. For those battling with the MYSD, use of cortisone over a period long enough to cause immune suppression is not a very good idea. While it may provide some short-term symptom relief, it is counterproductive in the long haul, leading to a fungal nightmare. This leaves the Jefferies protocol (discussed in the stress section), which theoretically does not involve immune suppressive doses of hydrocortisone (they are typically 5 mg doses four times per day). I have also found the use of cortisone nasal sprays or even excessive use of strong cortisone skin creams can aggravate yeast overgrowth and I avoid them. Other hormones, particularly progesterone, similarly encourage overgrowth, and women on birth control pills are known to be predisposed to yeast infections [198]. I also consider magnesium supplementation a very important part of the Candida protocol, since it is depleted by AH, leading to a further compromise of the immune system, as well as to gut problems [199].

The next part of the Candida control protocol is to make the gut somewhat inhospitable to fungal overgrowth, using the principal of competitive exclusion, discussed above in the dirt section. The objective is to fill many of the gut receptor sites that might be used by Candida with some friendly stuff that can adhere to these sites. At one time I thought that conventional probiotics could fill the bill, and it may work for many in controlling overgrowth. However, in the presence of mercury, it seems something stronger is necessary for this task. Enter dirt!

Of the two spore-former species I discussed above, bacillus laterosporus has a history of controlling Candida overgrowth in even the most difficult of cases. I routinely take one per day, and when detoxing with the Dirt Detox Protocol I am on a daily dose of two per day to assist in keeping the gut flora under control.

Now that we have added defense system support and competitive exclusion to the fungal protocol, let's move on to a discussion of antifungals themselves (fungicides that actually kill the fungus). Although I said we do not want to do any major Candida destruction to avoid mercury overload, it would be nice to have something available for gentle control. An ideal candidate would be a natural antifungal, which has MA's seal of approval on it for use in the human body, which is only toxic to the bad stuff, and is impervious to the development of resistance. Re-enter iodine!

Not only is iodine an excellent antifungal [200], it is also a detox agent, as we shall see in the halogen section below. To the extent that it liberates mercury by killing yeast, it may assist in pushing it out of the body (it is not a chelator). As a matter of interest, Dr. Truss, one of the first to identify the Candida problem in the 1950s, is said to have successfully used Lugol's solution as an antifungal agent, years before most of the pharmaceutical agents were available. He apparently prescribed 6 to 8 drops four times per day, which is about 150-200 milligrams per day, more than 1000 times the RDA of iodine.

As part of my halogen detox protocol, I routinely take 75 mg of iodine daily (with occasional breaks) which, along with the immune system boosting supplement ProBoost, has kept my Candida overgrowth under control without aggravating the mercury detox side effects. I have found that for Candida control, Lugol's solution is a better choice than iodine tablets. Some iodine tablets have an enteric coating so that they do not dissolve until they have passed the stomach. For Candida control, you may well want the iodine in the mouth, esophagus, and upper intestine, so I swish a diluted amount of it in the mouth, and sip it slowly to get the best effect. Recall that there are now two strengths of Lugol's solution on the market. The Truss formula used the original full-strength version, so adjustments should be made if the new reduced strength product is used. Regarding pre- and probiotics, it remains unclear if one or both of these products actually feed the multitude of fungal strains in the gut, so I would use caution until sufficient fungal and parasite detox has taken place.

To wrap up the Candida discussion, my analysis of the persistent Candida overgrowth problem is that it is intimately involved with mercury toxicity. Further, trying to wipe out Candida in this instance is counterproductive and actually not likely to be successful long term as long as mercury levels remain high. The defense system is sufficiently damaged by mercury that Candida overgrowth would quickly return even if you could temporarily wipe it out. I have outlined a protocol of defense system support (boosting the immune system and magnesium levels), competitive exclusion (using spore-formers), and mild antifungal use (iodine) to keep things under control. I believe this is a good overall approach to a very difficult detoxification problem involving many players. I continue to experiment with the Dirt Detox protocol to evaluate its role in controlling the fungal problem.

Before leaving the fungal area, I would like to mention the problem of mold, which is fungus gone wild. The mold problem, sometimes referred to as the "Sick Building Syndrome," usually originates in a home or building with insufficient ventilation and sunlight, and excess moisture, coupled with building materials that foster fungal growth. If the damage is sufficiently extensive, usually the only solution is total destruction. In this regard, I have some suggestions in the lifestyle section on living environment regarding home construction. Several books on mold toxicity have been written, and they indicate that supplements that bind with bile have been used with success in treating symptoms from mold exposure [201]. The use of apple pectin may be particularly useful in this instance. It is my belief that following The Wellness Project, including the suggestions in this section, will at least free up the defense system to deal with mold to the greatest extent possible.

The Bacterial Problem

In this section, we are going to visit the issue of toxic bacteria in the body, where it came from, and what to do about it. First, let's look at some of the history related to treatments for bacterial infections. The Germ Theory, promulgated by Pasteur, states that microorganisms are the cause of infections. This was in conflict with the Terrain Theory that said a compromised immune system causes infections. Claude Bernard and Antoine Bechamp popularized this theory in the mid 1800's [202]. One of the fundamental precepts of The Detox Plan is to strengthen the internal environment and in this regard, is in alignment with the Terrain Theory. This conflict of theories is yet another example where the medical community has confused necessary causes with sufficient causes. For an infection to occur requires both a pathogenic microorganism *and* a compromised defense system. Each is necessary, but neither in itself is sufficient to result in an infection. Therefore, I will now take the liberty of combining the Germ and Terrain Theories into what I will coin "The Infection Theory™," as follows: An infection requires a potentially pathogenic microorganism and a compromised defense system incapable of controlling the growth and dissemination of that organism.

We now read almost daily that the "Antibiotic Era" is fast coming to an end as bacteria mutate faster than we can create antibiotics, spawning deadly strains that are resistant to everything Big Pharma has to offer. (As you will see, The Detox Plan has a "secret weapon" for these critters, courtesy of MA).

Our intestinal bacteria, sometimes referred to as the microflora or microbiome, plays a very big role in keeping us healthy, and it is a very important part of our defense system. A goal of Nature's Detox Plan is to support the body to establish or reestablish a healthy gut environment, and the suggested soil components play an important role. Enter mercury again.

In spite of all the negative things I have said about mercury, it is a very potent antibiotic and antifungal, and for many years was the preferred medication to treat syphilis. While it sometimes cured the disease, many times it killed the patient. Now, let's think about this: there is finally general consensus, even by the ADA (American Dental

Association), that amalgam fillings outgas mercury continuously into the body. If mercury is an antibiotic, theoretically, those with amalgams in place have a built-in lifetime source of antibiotics leaking into their body 24/7. Sounds good, but it is not.

There has been a lot of press lately on how the over-prescription of antibiotics has spawned super-bacteria such as MRSA (methicillin resistant staphylococcus aureus) and other nasty flesh-eating stuff. The problem, of course, is that bacteria are able to become resistant to antibiotics when exposed to them long enough. Further, we know that taking antibiotics, which do not discriminate between good and bad gut bacteria, kills virtually everything, leaving a person vulnerable to regrowth of what could be a very unbalanced mix of flora. Can you image what a lifetime of mercury infusion has done to gut flora? A few bright scientists have undertaken the study of this issue and have found that mercury has not only spawned a host of mercury-resistant bacteria, but that most of these strains have also acquired the traits of resistance to antibiotics in general [203] [204] [205] [206]. If you never had any amalgams, could you still end up with these Frankenbacteria? Well, a group of children was tested who never had amalgam restorations, but who had presumably been vaccinated with thimerosal. They were found to harbor bacteria that were both mercury and general antibiotic resistant [207].

Other than the usual industry denials regarding the above, it is not rocket science to see we have a serious issue here. Considering the number of people that have been exposed to mercury via amalgams or vaccines, I am not sure there are many walking around with what could be called "normal" gut flora. Unless this is accounted for, it would seem that the NIH gut bacteria study might come to the wrong conclusion as to what should be used for a blueprint for healthy gut flora, especially if they do not also account for spore-forming bacteria missing in virtually everyone's gut. From personal experience and other anecdotal reports, I can tell you that mercury can severely influence digestive function by altering gut bacteria, causing what is called intestinal dysbiosis, and making it somewhat impossible to achieve the desired bowel characteristics described in the defecation section above. Symptoms can range from oral thrush (mouth fungus), to GERD, to halitosis, to gut pain, to IBS, to IBD (Irritable Bowel Disease), to constipation, to diarrhea, and to nutrient deficiencies in general. From my point of view, the long-term solution is to follow *The Original Diet* and *Nature's Detox Plan* to get rid of mercury. Spore-forming bacteria play a critical role in restoring gut function.

Just when you thought we were done with dental issues and bacteria problems, along come root canals, which I refer to as toxic time bombs. A fellow member of the Advisory Board of the Price-Pottenger Nutrition Foundation was Dr. George Meinig, a retired dentist with an extensive career in the field of endodontistry, a sub-specialty dealing with tooth root and pulp issues, including the root canal procedure. Early in his career, Dr. Meinig pioneered in root canal procedures, and was one of the founders of what is now the American Association of Endodontics, who have conferred upon him honorary recognition for his work in the field. When he spoke on the subject of root canals, I listened very carefully. During his career, he became interested in the work of Weston Price, a dentist himself, and by perusing the archives at the Price-Pottenger Nutrition Foundation, discovered reams of research by Price on root canals, documents that had been suppressed by the dental community beginning over 70 years ago. What came out of his research was a book entitled *The Root Canal Cover-up* by George E. Meinig DDS FACD [208] which should be read by everyone who has ever had a root canalled tooth or is contemplating one.

What Price found and Meinig brought to light was that virtually all root-canalled teeth were loaded with bacteria that were producing toxins, and that the toxins were able to travel down the tooth canal to virtually all parts of the body. While a strong defense system is usually able to keep the toxins in check, it just takes some precipitating event that drags down the defense system to enable the toxins to cause major illness. In a fascinating series of experiments, Price was able to take an extracted root-canalled tooth from an ill patient, implant it under the skin of a rabbit, and cause the same illness in the rabbit. Price's studies were conducted over a 25-year period, included a team of 60 scientists, filled 1174 pages, and were conducted under the auspices of the American Dental Association. Unfortunately, some members of that organization decided to bury the results. They also refused to accept the focal theory of infection, where a primary infection can cause systemic illness. We saw this issue resurface in the Candida discussion.

The root canal problem is really not rocket science. There are miles of microtubules that run throughout every tooth. Once a root canal procedure has been performed, the tooth is dead and the blood supply is cut off, so there is no way for the body to control the contents of these tubules, which are filled with bacteria that cannot be reached by antibiotics or anything else. Over time (actually, your lifetime) these bacteria produce virulent toxins that leak down through the tooth canal and, but for the constant vigilance of the defense system, are capable of making the patient ill. Dentists place *gutta percha*, a latex discovered about 150 years ago and derived from the sap of trees grown in Asia, into the opening they made in the tooth when they filed out the pulp, in the hope that it will seal up the opening. Typically, it does not, so more bacteria seeps into the dead tooth.

Recently, new procedures have been tried to fix the problem, but so far there is no proof that they work any better. One is to use a laser to try to sterilize the miles of tubules, and then to use calcium hydroxide (Biocalex® is one brand) as a filler. Approaches that are more recent use ozone and/or oxygen to try to sterilize the tooth. As pointed out in the book *The Roots of Disease* by Robert Kulacz, DDS and Thomas Levy, MD, JD [209], neither the laser nor ozone nor calcium hydroxide do the job. If you are unsure whether your root-canalled teeth are currently toxic, there is a simple and inexpensive test to provide you and your dentist with some answers. It is called the TOPAS test (Toxicity Prescreening Assay), and is available as a research tool to participating dentists [210] while it awaits regulatory approval in the US.

From the perspective of rocket science, root canal procedures are really a technological failure, and would never get you off the launching pad. I share the opinions of Drs. Meinig, Kulacz, Levy and many others that the procedure does not work as intended and has the potential of making someone quite ill. Nevertheless, just like in the diet studies, there is no doubt in my mind that there are folks who can live to 100 in perfect health with a mouth full of root canals. Undoubtedly, they have been endowed with a very strong defense system, and have succeeded in avoiding any catastrophes in life that might impair it. Are you one of them? If not, and if you have root-canalled teeth and wish to keep them, it would be prudent not get sick. The illness list caused by root canal toxins is heavily biased towards heart disease, and the above referenced books have long lists of many other illnesses, which cover virtually everything imaginable.

Root canals are in second place, just behind amalgams, on my list of the major technology errors in the fields of dentistry and medicine. I do applaud the endodontist community for trying hard to find a solution to the problem with new technologies. In the meanwhile, if you have an irreparably damaged tooth, as I did, I believe the safe option is extraction, with a permanent bridge replacement. I have given copies of the above referenced books on root canal issues to friends who have mentioned they are going in for a root canal procedure. Among those who read them, all opted for extraction. Ah, now we get to extractions – and you thought we were finished with the dental industry. Onward to cavitations.

A cavitation is a hole or defect in the jawbone at the site of an old or healed tooth extraction. It may also be present around an infected tooth such as a root canal-treated tooth. The contents of a cavitation typically consist of highly toxic and infected bone and dead tissue, essentially identical in appearance to gangrene as seen in other parts of the body. Studies done with people that have had wisdom tooth extractions show that most have cavitations at these old extraction sites. Many cavitations form when the bone surrounding an extracted tooth is not properly cleansed and treated prior to the closing of the wound.

Procedures for doing this have been developed, and Hal Huggins, mentioned above, has a referral list of oral surgeons trained to perform them. As far as diagnostic tools for detecting cavitations, a trained dentist can use either finger feel, or pin pressure on the bone, or the TOPAS test mentioned above. An even more elegant method is to use ultrasound to view the upper and lower jawbone for cavitation detection. A popular device for accomplishing this is the Cavitat®, and many specially trained oral surgeons use this device [211] because cavitations are sometimes difficult to find, and rarely produce fever or other such signs of infection. In addition to a boatload of illnesses, cavitations are well known for producing facial and other upper body pain, and cleaning them out can remove symptoms almost instantly. I strongly suggest that everyone who has had extractions or root canals be tested at least once for cavitations.

Moving out of the mouth, while there are a plethora of bacteria surrounding us (many of them found in hospitals), one group in particular deserves special attention because of their persistence. These bacteria cause the condition known as Lyme disease, an infectious disease that has stirred up a huge controversy in the medical community, who are busy arguing over the definition. It's clear to me though, and to many doctors, that this is a quite real, serious, and under-diagnosed disease, which can have life-altering consequences, and may be contagious. The disease is believed to be caused by bacteria from the genus *Borrelia* and is transmitted to humans by the bite of infected insects. Symptoms often include fever, headache, fatigue, and sometimes a typical skin rash. The fatigue is bad enough to keep you in bed, and other symptoms, including arthritic-like joint pain, can be disabling.

Officially, the thinking is that most early cases can be treated with large doses of antibiotics for a few weeks. If not caught quickly, some experts advocate massive doses of antibiotics for several years, while others admit that they have not figured out a cure. Dr. Klinghardt has spent many years looking for treatment strategies, and the results of his work can be found in the protocol section of his website [34]. There are interesting parallels between some of the symptoms of Lyme and mercury toxicity, as well as similarities to parasite infestation, and even autism [212]. There is a fascinating protocol in the parasite section below that has given relief to many Lyme sufferers.

To gain control over some of these nasty bacteria as part of a detox program, I have a few natural suggestions. The first is the spore-forming bacteria, for all of the reasons previously mentioned. I have experimented with getting these bacteria into the body by means of nasal sprays, eardrops, skin sprays, and gargles, all with good results. There is no magic formula; I simply put some spore-former powder, say from two capsules, in an ounce or two of mineral water, and put it into a suitable dispenser. I have also added a capsule of humic/fulvic acid to the mix. As far as oral intake, I have experimented with very large spore-former doses (up to 20 capsules per day) for several weeks with no ill effects. An interesting research project would be to treat Lyme suffers with saturation doses of spore-formers to see if they can competitively eliminate or even kill the Borrelia bacteria.

There are many herbal remedies to ward off bacterial infections, and each has a niche. One in particular is somewhat broad-based, and comes from nature's arsenal of plant protectors. It is the seed and pulp of grapefruit, which one would not normally eat because these portions of fruit are naturally toxic. If you are ill or going to be exposed to infections, grapefruit seed extract (GSE), not to be confused with grape seed extract, is a product that has proved helpful, and is widely available as a liquid or tablet. Another herb discussed more fully below is artemesia.

Then there is the latest favorite in non-prescription antibiotics – colloidal silver. As you can tell from some of the earlier discussions in this book, I have done a fair amount of research into silver, which, by the way, can be classified as a heavy metal, is not believed to be an essential mineral, and is known to be toxic at very high exposures. There are many safe colloidal products on the market, and I will tell you about my favorite in a moment. First, some potentially bad news about silver, which, strangely enough, takes us back to amalgam fillings. If you remember, amalgams are about 50% mercury and 50% *silver*. Well, silver does not outgas like mercury, but you can bet that a lifetime of silver in your mouth has caused a certain amount of silver, through abrasion, diffusion, and other processes, to be floating around your body 24/7, and certainly, there would be a very high concentration in the mouth. Could it be that this has spawned silver-resistant bacteria, just as mercury has spawned mercury-resistant bacteria? Apparently so.

A small study conducted on bacteria found on teeth with amalgam fillings identified bacteria strains that were both silver-resistant and also generally resistant to prescription antibiotics [213]. A survey of silver-resistant bacteria shows that several are starting to pop up, which is quite unfortunate. Silver coatings are used widely as microbials in medical procedures, including those involving the insertion of catheters and stents. For the most part, however, silver still has a good track record, and I suggest the brand Sovereign Silver® made by Natural-Immunogenics Corp. [214]. To avoid developing a resistance, I would only use silver sparingly as needed. Alcohol and chlorine are other candidates for antibacterials, but both are toxic. Wouldn't it be great if there was a natural antibiotic, which has MA's seal of approval on it for use in the human body, and (so far) is impervious to the development of resistance? Enter iodine!

I have discussed iodine previously as a detox agent and a potent and natural antibiotic that is also an essential mineral. As far as I am concerned, it is a powerhouse in the category of natural antibiotics. When one studies the literature, there are essentially no reports of any significance showing iodine-resistant bacteria other than an anecdotal report or two. This is good news indeed, since as anyone who has had a hospital medical procedure performed at a hospital is aware, iodine is the antibacterial of choice to clean wounds as well as the surgeon's hands. Speaking of hand cleaning, the many varieties of antibacterial soaps on the market usually contain triclosan as the active ingredient. Reports are starting to surface that widespread use of these products may be creating antibiotic-resistant strains of bacteria, and I avoid their use. My choice for hand cleaners are those containing iodine, including povidone-iodine topical antiseptics such as the line of Betadine® products by Purdue Pharma [215], or the many generic products including swabs, sprays and other items listed under povidone or povidone-iodine and sold at most drugstores.

Iodine in the form of Lugol's solution can also be used topically, but it does stain the skin, so one might want to try the Clayodine compound mentioned above. Using iodine topically may well result in systemic absorption, and symptoms of detoxification may arise. For use as a systemic antibiotic, I would take several drops of Lugol's solution in fruit tea and/or gargle with the diluted solution, or take one or more Iodoral tablets. For further discussion, see the halogen section below.

One cannot discuss bacteria without revisiting conventional probiotics. In the discussion in the diet section, I mentioned that probiotics could be helpful or harmful, depending on who benefits more from them, you or the bad guys in your gut. As you can see from the detox discussion so far, there are plenty of bad guys, and there are more to come. My suggestion stands of taking modest doses of only a few strains, at least until a detox program has had a chance to decrease the critter load, which not only includes bacteria, but also fungi and parasites, all of which might indirectly benefit from a large dose of pre- and probiotics. This note of caution arises from my personal experiments, where, based on symptoms, I was able to worsen Candida overgrowth by taking large doses of conventional probiotics. Others have also found that probiotics can feed parasites [216], and prebiotics such as FOS can feed unwelcome bacteria, especially *Klebsiella pneumoniae, hemolytic E. coli, Bacteroides* species, and *Staphylococcus aureus* [217].

This note of caution does not apply to spore-formers, which do not suffer any of the problems associated with conventional probiotics, and that brings me to a discussion of the Dirt Detox Protocol as applied to bacteria. Spore-formers such as bacillus laterosporus have been tested against salmonella and pathogenic strains of E. coli with excellent results, so I would expect the protocol to work well against toxic gut bacteria.

Regarding testing for nasty gut bacteria, there are a number of stool tests that can be performed that may be useful in analyzing gut bacteria, fungi, and parasites. One that I have used is called the CDSA (Comprehensive Digestive Stool Analysis) test by Genova Diagnostics [218].

The Parasite Problem

Closely allied to the fungal problem is the parasite problem. For purposes of this section, I will define parasites as including worms, amoeba, flukes, and protozoa. Like bacteria and fungi, most parasites reside in our gut, and some are friendly while others are not. Also like bacteria and fungi, we have yet to identify what are probably thousands of different parasites in our gut. Many folks deny they have parasites, but in my opinion, it is virtually impossible to avoid them whenever you open your mouth and put something in it, and they may also enter via the eyes, ears, nose, and skin. I feel comfortable making the statement that virtually everyone who has not been routinely treated for them harbors parasites. At present and for the foreseeable future, it is practically impossible to prove me wrong because there is no foolproof test for parasite infestation, and I have tried many. Obviously, it is hard to test for strains of parasites we have yet to identify, but there is no lack of trying by a multitude of test labs.

We can get many clues about parasites from the animal kingdom (including insects), where this issue is taken very seriously, as it should be.

Animals spend a great deal of time managing their parasite infestations and they are highly attuned to know when they are infected. Humans, on the other hand, know virtually nothing about parasites and have lost any instinct regarding whether or not we are infested. Clues from MA such as intestinal discomfort are treated with the usual symptom-suppressing OTC and prescription products, without getting to the source of the problem. For this reason, most of us are walking around with a lifetime load of untreated parasite infestations for which the symptom list goes on for pages. To find clues to infestation, let's look at how animals deal with the problem, as explained in Cindy Engel's book *Wild Health*, a major source of the following information [3].

For parasite control, most animals resort to the toxins in the parts of plants that we avoid as food choices in *The Original Diet*. In their war against parasites, they choose plants that are not part of their normal diet, usually very bitter, and whose levels of toxicity can sometimes approach lethal amounts. They will also eat rough plant parts, mostly folded leaves, in an effort to hook on to and scrape parasites from the intestinal wall, known as the Velcro® effect. Dogs and cats are occasionally known to eat grass, which can have a scouring effect as well as promote vomiting as an additional purge. Actually, tolerance of or a desire for very bitter plants, even in humans, has been directly correlated with the degree of parasite infestation in that person, and as the infestation decreases, so does the tolerance of bitters. The bitters usually include tannins, saponins and other alkaloids toxic to parasites. The plant *vernonia amygdalina* is particularly potent, and studies are underway to investigate its use as a drug.

Another way in which animals control parasites is through the purgative effect of *salt*. Parasite infested camels routinely seek out the very salty plant *Salvadora persica*_(commonly known as peelu), as well as salt-rich wells to gain the purging effects of salt. As you will see below, I view this as a major clue from MA regarding parasite control. Yet another animal control method for parasites is our old friend clay. It appears to help in three ways: by adsorbing toxins excreted by the parasites, by physically expelling worm eggs, and by protecting the gut from invasion from migrating worm larvae [219]. Before going into a discussion on parasite control, a caution is warranted on the use of pre- or probiotics when a heavy parasite load may be present, because they may well end up feeding the parasites. Once clearance has occurred, then some higher-dose, broader-strain products might be helpful [216] [220].

So far, from our excursion into the animal world we have discovered that toxic plant parts, clay, and salt are all used as natural remedies. I suggest these same routes for human parasite cleansing. Starting with plant parts, there are many herbal parasite-cleanse products on the market, and here are some of the protocols I have used with good results. The first is an herbal concoction that has been used for many years, and is produced and sold directly by a small company called Humaworm, Inc. [221]. It is a 30-day program of two capsules per day, which can be repeated every 90 days, if necessary. Their website lists the formula, and has some helpful information regarding symptoms and detox reactions. Generally, every six months I repeat the cleanse.

The second suggestion is known as the Clark Para-Cleanse protocol, using green-black walnut hulls, wormwood (artemesia), and common cloves. The ingredients and one-week protocol for using them are widely available in health food stores and on the web. The black walnut hulls and wormwood kill adult and developmental stages of many types of parasites, and the cloves kill the eggs. This protocol is high dose/short time, and can produce some unexpectedly severe die-off reactions such as dizziness and nausea, so you might want to have a partner around during the program. This protocol can also be repeated once every several months. When you have cleaned out everything that these formulas are able to handle, you should notice no symptoms upon redoing the protocol. None of these formulas is perfect, and they are not capable of removing all forms of parasites, so let's move on to clay .

The types of clay and dosages previously mentioned as part of the Dirt Detox Protocol may be incorporated into an herbal parasite cleanse, or even delayed until immediately thereafter. Remember to separate the taking of clay and other soil components from the herbs by about two hours.

At this point, I would like to mention the problem of pollution-linked illnesses involving parasitic organisms, many of which are acquired by eating seafood from polluted waters. Books have been written on this topic [222] and it is my belief that following The Wellness Project, including the suggestions in this book, will at least free up the defense system to deal with this problem to the extent possible.

Now for the real surprise in the human world of parasite cleansing – salt. If we had paid more attention to the animal world in the past, perhaps the role of salt as a parasite cleanser would have surfaced sooner. A few years ago, a group of Lyme disease sufferers tried an experiment of taking large doses of salt (eight grams or more per day) along with vitamin C. What happened next was quite unexpected – parasites of all sorts started to exit their bodies in great numbers from unusual locations such as their eyes, ears, and skin. As a result of this discovery, the Salt/C protocol, as it is called, was launched. Some long-time Lyme sufferers who were getting nowhere with conventional treatment suddenly found major relief using this protocol. A website has been launched showing photos of many types of parasites that have exited bodies, and I caution the reader that some of these photos can be quite unsettling [223]. While the experiments so far have been primarily with Lyme sufferers, there is no reason to suppose this protocol will not work for anyone suffering from parasites for whatever reason. It does raise the question, however, as to whether the insect bite or sting that transfers the Lyme bacteria may also be transferring parasites directly into the bloodstream, which then spread everywhere and rapidly multiply.

From the website, you can find the details of the protocol. There are web support forums for those experimenting with it (look for Yahoo groups with the word *lyme* in the title). For my own experiments, I used ancient seabed unrefined salt, mentioned earlier, and put it into 00 size gelatin capsules. I also used buffered vitamin C capsules and took up to ten grams per day of both for a few weeks. Because I had done extensive parasite cleanses beforehand, I had no surprises. By the way, the objective of these protocols is not necessarily to totally eradicate all parasites from the body. Some studies have shown that having a small amount hanging around may be beneficial for some intestinal illnesses [224].

The dramatic effects of salt as a natural detoxifier (even more on this in the next section) raises the question of whether our low-salt craze, which has been recently escalated to a near hysterical anti-salt movement, has jeopardized the health of millions by essentially eliminating this natural defender. This is not rocket science. I don't think it is a coincidence that MA has provided us with salt taste buds, or that the blood of our prey contains pounds of salt. Here is one more of my predictions. The low-salt craze will eventually make it to the top-ten list of technology blunders in the history of medicine. This brings me to a discussion of bromide.

The Halogen Problem

I have already acquainted the reader with iodine (a halogen) as a detoxifier, so let's look at what there is left to detoxify (plenty). Iodine's toxic halogen cousins that are of interest to us are the bromides, fluorides and a chlorine compound known as perchlorate. Let's start with bromine, and bromide, which is a reduced form of bromine. Bromine may or may not be an essential micromineral in the body in extremely small doses, but in excess it is very bad news, and we are awash in it. Currently, bromide is found in pesticides (methyl bromide); bread products (potassium bromate); brominated vegetable oil that may be added to citrus-flavored drinks; hot tub disinfectants; certain asthma inhalers and prescription drugs; personal care products like toothpaste and mouthwash; fabric dyes; and as flame retardants (PBDEs) in drapes, coats, pajamas, mattresses, carpeting, and most plastic products in consumer applications such as computers and cell phones.

As reported in Dr. Brownstein's book on iodine, previously cited [124], bromine in sufficient concentrations replaces iodine in the body. The results: every thyroid condition you can think of, including hypo- and hyperthyroid and autoimmune conditions to thyroid cancer; skin conditions known as bromoderma, which can express as acne-like lesions, cherry angiomas and other strange rashes; mental conditions from depression to schizophrenia; hearing problems; and kidney cancer from bromates such as those used as dough conditioners in bread products. This last application is another technology blunder that should be recognized with some sort of award.

Dough conditioners are used to increase production of bread-making, in other words, to save money. Originally, iodine compounds were used in this application, but because of an erroneous conclusion that consumers would ingest excessive iodine, in the 1980s the industry switched over to potassium bromate, a known carcinogen. This substance is banned in Canada and the UK, but is considered safe in the U.S. Fortunately for The Original Diet users, we dodge this blunder.

Are there any clues from MA substantiating the bromine debacle? Yes, a very sad one. A recent study was conducted in an attempt to find the causes of an epidemic among cats of feline hyperthyroidism (FH). Brominated flame retardants known as polybrominated diphenyl ethers (PBDEs) came up as a major culprit [225]. Pet cats may be like canaries in coalmines when it comes to evaluating the health impacts of these persistent chemicals, used in carpets, furniture, and electronics. Veterinarians first noticed a dramatic surge in feline hyperthyroidism (FH) in the 1980s, coinciding with the use of PBDEs as flame-retardants in consumer products. FH, the most common endocrine disorder in cats, causes rapid weight loss due to increased concentrations of thyroxine. They found that hyperthyroidal cats had very high body burdens of PBDEs, which are in residential carpeting as well as in cat food, particularly fish-flavored canned brands. Cats swallow PBDEs in food and by licking PBDE-laden house dust from their fur. The bromine atoms in the PBDEs mimic the iodine in thyroxine, displacing it and leading to the FH condition. The potential link between FH and PBDEs suggests that house cats may be sentinels for chronic indoor PBDE exposure in people. As the author of the study speculated, "like cats, toddlers may be inordinately exposed to PBDEs in dust by crawling on floors and placing objects in their mouths."

Wherever you are currently reading this book, the odds are that you are surrounded by this bromine-laden chemical, since it is in most upholstered furniture and in plastic enclosures for electrical and electronic products. Perhaps the human epidemic of subclinical hypothyroidism (bromine can cause hypo- or hyperthyroid conditions) is related to these chemicals, which are also found in high concentrations in lake, river and farmed fish. Even worse, fish also contain PCBs, and a study has shown the combination of the two (PBDEs and PCBs) interact in a manner that enhances their individual neurotoxicity [226].

The cat study mentioned above prompts me to suggest another clue from MA. If you have pets and they are exhibiting illness, perhaps you are at risk, since you share the same environment. As you will see in the lifestyle section, I am not in favor of indoor carpeting, and this is one more reason for my position. While we are on the subject of thyroid glands, there are many studies linking thyroid conditions to deranged cholesterol levels, particularly elevated LDL levels, so the halogen problem may extend its tentacles all the way into the statin drug arena [227].

Under certain conditions, bromide in water may be converted to bromate, a known carcinogen, if ozone is used in the water purification cycle. This has led to some embarrassments for the bottled water industry (a large recall), as well as for the Los Angeles Water Department, who recently announced the dumping of 600 million gallons of bromate-contaminated water, possibly as the result of ozonation of bromide contaminated water. It also seems possible that bromide in the presence of chlorine and sunlight can be converted to bromates. Some forms of charcoal, and RO water filters remove bromates.

Using bromine (or chlorine) for hot tub or swimming pool disinfection is definitely not a good idea, and I suggest ozone instead as the best of the alternatives, notwithstanding the bromate conversion problem I just mentioned. The solution is to start with bromide-free water, and then the bromate conversion problem is moot. Knowledgeable ozone system manufacturers can design pool and spa systems to minimize such conversion. One ozone system manufacturer that I have used is Clearwater Tech LLC, in San Luis Obispo, California [228].

Because bromine interferes with iodine and is so ubiquitous, it may well be a major player in what seems to be an epidemic of thyroid illnesses. Earlier in this book, I discussed my theory regarding autoimmune diseases, pointing to toxins as the ultimate culprit. Two prevalent autoimmune conditions involve the thyroid gland and are named Graves' disease and Hashimoto's disease. Dr. Brownstein has found that proper treatment with iodine can reduce or eliminate the symptoms related to both of these conditions. I believe this occurs because iodine displaces the toxic halogens from occupying iodine receptor sites, and when this occurs, the defense system no longer treats the thyroid cells as foreign. I see no reason why this cannot also apply to the other autoimmune conditions.

In addition to the thyroid gland, recent studies have identified iodine as a critically important element in virtually all of the organs of the body, including the ovaries and mammary glands of women, leading to speculation that bromine may also be a contributor to breast and ovarian diseases, including cancer. Bromine is not the only player in the list of halogen elements that interfere with the body's use of iodine. Enter fluoride.

The health police deliberately put fluoride, a form of fluorine, into our drinking water, supposedly to prevent dental carries. That is almost as irrational as putting mercury in our mouths, and certainly deserves a high place of honor in the technology-blunder hall of fame. Books have been written on this blunder [229], and an article in *Scientific American* offers a good summary of the issues [230]. In a nutshell, not only does fluoride not achieve its objective of reducing tooth decay in children (who mostly drink soda!), it poisons the entire community. By now, it should be well known that the dental benefit of fluoride, if any, is only topical, not systemic; the toxic effects of fluoride are sufficiently severe that regulatory agencies caution against making infant formula with fluoridated water, and there is a poison warning on fluoridated toothpaste. Even the FDA will not approve fluoridated water as safe or effective because there is no evidence that it is.

The effects of excess fluoride include weakened bone strength and bone cancer, brain damage, tooth discoloration, decreased thyroid function, and the constellation of illnesses surrounding the interference with iodine. Years ago, fluoride was actually used to treat hyperthyroidism, because of its ability to interfere with iodine. It also interferes with the absorption of magnesium [10], which is already in short supply for most people and is needed to build strong teeth! As the reader by now knows, and as the studies of Weston Price and PA skeletal evidence have shown, tooth decay is prevented by following the correct diet, one that is in alignment with our heritage. I have already discussed water filtration for those unfortunate enough to live in a fluoridated community, and I would add to that the avoidance of any product containing fluoride, including toothpaste, most SSRI antidepressants, fluoroquinolone-based antibiotics, dental bonding agents, and some nasal sprays. More details are available at the Fluoride Action Network [231].

Chlorine and perchlorate round out the toxic halogen family, all of which interfere with iodine. The elimination of chlorine in drinking and bathing water was discussed above in the water filter section.

Perchlorates, which used to be used as a thyroid depressing medication, are used modernly as a rocket fuel, and are also found in car airbags and fireworks. They also have contaminated many of our wells and rivers. Vegetables such as lettuce contain high amounts from irrigation water, as does cow and breast milk.

The protocols to offset the halogen problems listed above are not rocket science. Reduce your exposure to the toxic halogens, and increase your intake of iodine, which acts to displace the other halogens and take their place. The iodine testing and supplementation procedures have already been covered. I personally have been taking large doses of iodine daily for some time, so perhaps relating my experiences would be helpful. Shortly after beginning a daily dose of 25 mg of iodine, skin problems characteristic of bromine excretion began to appear on my face. Others undergoing this protocol have reported redness, rashes, and pustules around the "butterfly" area of the face – over the nose and cheeks. In my case, the rash was slightly above this area, across my eyebrows and the bridge of my nose, and including the area above my eyelids, forming an exact outline of my sinuses. It resolved within two weeks. However, when I increased the dose to 50 mg, the rashes reappeared, only to resolve again a few weeks later.

I have repeated this process several times and as of the writing of this book, I am up to 75 mg, and the bromine (and probably fluoride and perchlorates) continues to be excreted through my skin. While this process is annoying, I feel good that I am getting rid of a lifetime of this stuff, so I put up with it. Anecdotal reports by clinicians experimenting on themselves and measuring bromine excretion from their bodies indicate that the process may continue for several years, a testament to our lifetime exposure. Because rashes can detract from our appearance, others and I have experimented with cosmetic cover-ups for use during the detox process. Mineral-based powders are a candidate if they do not contain any toxic minerals such as aluminum or titanium, and do not use nano-particles, which increase absorption. If you use a moisturizer (discussed more fully in the lifestyle section), apply the powder over it to minimize the chances of absorption. There is more about safe and natural cosmetics in the lifestyle section.

Through continued experimentation, researchers have found that our old friend salt, in combination with vitamin C, can be used as part of the halogen detox protocol to improve results in some recalcitrant cases [232]. I believe this discovery occurred independently from the salt/C protocol used in connection with parasite cleansing, and I wonder how many more applications we may uncover for this unusual duet. For those readers with a further interest, there are support- and research-oriented groups online that discuss these iodine protocols (look for Yahoo groups with the word *iodine* in their name).

Lastly, the Dirt Detox Protocol may be of benefit in treating the halogen problem. There have been reports of urine alkalization alone having been used successfully to treat fluoride toxicity [46], and I suspect alkalization will speed up the removal of other halogens. Please don't think we are done with the halogen discussion. Wait until we get to the discussion of lighting in the lifestyle section to revisit bromine – think *halogen* lamps.

The Virus Problem

Viruses are in the news on a regular basis, from AIDS to the constellation of herpes family viruses (oral, genital, shingles), along with the new vaccines for shingles and the human papilloma virus. A relatively new field of scientific investigation known as Paleovirology has undertaken the task of understanding the role of viruses in our genetic heritage, and reports are starting to emerge on the findings from these studies [233]. The researchers have found in our DNA the fragments of long-vanished viruses that probably have been with us for our entire evolutionary history. The supposition is that viruses have been and always will be part of our heritage, and may actually have acted - and will continue to act - to shape our genetic future. My understanding from this is that we are loaded with viruses. Once they have infected us, they are likely to hang around for a lifetime, and our sole defense is our defense system. This is in alignment with my objective in The Wellness Project to do whatever is possible to keep the defense system from being burdened with the wrong foods and other toxins, so that it can deal with important stuff like viruses. Regarding the use of the Dirt Detox Protocol for viral issues, the soil components of fulvic/humic acids and spore-formers have both exhibited antiviral properties. I suggest trying topical as well as oral application of these soil compounds for those with viral outbreaks.

Many years ago, a good friend of mine was plagued with repeated oral herpes outbreaks, and I decided to do some research to see if I could find something to help. What came out of my research were two patents (which I have since donated to the public) for a topical method of exposing the herpes virus to the defense system so that it could more promptly suppress the outbreaks. Please see the separate side box labeled "Viruses and a Topically Applied Food Preservative" for more details.

Viruses and a Topically Applied Food Preservative

When the book *Life Extension* [234] came out more than 20 years ago, one of the fascinating topics discussed was the oral use of a widely-used artificial food preservative known as BHT (butylated hydroxytoluene) to suppress herpes simplex eruptions. I read everything I could on the subject and was not comfortable suggesting oral use of BHT to anyone because of the conflicting data on toxicity, ranging from non-toxic and health-promoting to possible toxicity issues [235]. I began experiments with the topical application of BHT bound to various lipids as a way around the potential toxicity issues, and settled on the combination of BHT mixed with Tea Tree Oil. Friends who tried it as a topical preparation achieved good results in suppressing or speeding up the healing of eruptions. My guess as to how it works is that the BHT dissolves the lipid outer layer of the virus, and the tea tree oil destroys what is left. I received two patents on the preparation, which I have since donated to the public, so that anyone is free to experiment with the idea. For those interested, see for example U.S. Patent 5,215,478 for more information [236].

It is well known that many types of viruses, including those in the herpes family, thrive on the amino acid arginine, and one of the simple protocols sufferers have used in the past is either to avoid arginine rich foods, which just happen to be nuts and seeds, or to take large doses of the competing amino acid lysine.

The EMF Problem

EMF (Electromagnetic Field) radiation toxicity is a hot topic today, involving everything from power lines to cell phones. I have done some research in the area, and looked for some simple protocols that can be implemented in an effort to reduce the risk of harm. Because of the long interval of time between cause and effect, it has been difficult to draw firm conclusions as to which type of radiation causes what condition, and to postulate safe levels of exposure. Therefore, the best approach is to minimize exposure.

Starting with electric field exposure, this issue typically arises in the home (and office), where we are surrounded with miles of wiring, located inside and outside of the walls, which are connected to the 60 Hz AC power system. The effect of this wiring on the body can be measured easily using a digital meter with an AC millivolt scale. Such meters are readily available, and one source is *lessemf.com* [237], which is a website that also provides many reference and educational resources that can be useful in this complicated arena. I am going to give you the short version.

Electric fields cause the buildup of an electrical charge on the human body relative to the earth, and this can be measured in AC volts. To eliminate this charge is not rocket science. All that needs to be done is electrically to connect your body to the earth, discharging the charge. Of course, PA had no problem with this for several reasons. First, he was not surrounded by electrical wires, and second he/she walked barefoot on native soil, placing him/her in electrical contact with the earth so no charge could have accumulated under any conditions. Well, the goal here is to emulate PA by reproducing the body/native soil connection in our lives as often as possible.

As it turns out, a whole industry was developed about 30 years ago to do just that, and I was a participant in its genesis way back then. At that time, using what is called the CMOS (Complementary Metal Oxide Semiconductor) process, electronic devices were being developed that were acutely sensitive to static charge. One annoying form of this with which we are all familiar is the voltage that accumulates on the body in dry weather and causes "shocks" when we touch a conductor. Well, such discharges also wipe out sensitive electronic parts, so all kinds of products were developed then to connect anyone working around electronics to earth. The industry is called the static control industry and includes wristbands, floor mats, seat pads, table coverings, special shoe and sock bindings, and electrically conductive clothing and packaging materials, all still widely available and in use today. These products employ all sorts of materials such as conductive fibers like silver or carbon that are coated on or woven into fabric. I made great use of these devices in the 1970s, where entire assembly lines of folks were grounded while working on electronic parts. For safety sake, we used resistors in the ground wiring to reduce the potential for shock.

The health benefits of grounding the body are recently being re-investigated, and some believe that it reduces inflammation and has a calming effect. If so, all of those grounded assembly workers have been indirectly getting a health benefit! For those interested in grounding themselves, it is simple to do so using these anti-static devices. The *lessemf.com* website has dozens of such items available, along with special cords to connect you to earth ground through house wiring. One company in particular, called Earth FX [238], is the source of specially designed mattress pads and sheets that can be used to connect you to earth while you sleep, and my wife and I have used one of their pads for some time. I also gave several to friends, some of whom claim they sleep better using them. Their website also lists some of the reported health benefits from using the pads, and they appear to have some patents for their pad designs.

As I mentioned above in connection with the use of FIR saunas, I believe there may be benefit to grounding oneself while inside. My interest is in the possibility that a charged body may interfere with the excretion of toxins. I am unaware of any research in this area, but I do feel better when grounded in the sauna. You can just use one of the many kinds of conductive wrist straps available, and a suitable wire out the door or vent of the sauna to a local AC ground connection. All commercial wrist straps contain a built-in safety resistor. A patent application has been filed covering this idea.

Summarizing the electric field discussion, the idea is to emulate PA, who was connected electrically to the earth by walking barefoot on moist soil or grass. We no longer are grounded because we usually walk with rubber or plastic shoes on cement, all of which are insulators. We have no path to discharge electrical energy that builds up on our bodies from all the gadgets and lights in our electrical surroundings, with unknown health effects. Obviously, to the extent possible, we should walk barefoot on earth or a beach. Barring that, there are many ways to hook yourself up inside the house.

Now, let's move on to magnetic fields, where cell phones are in the spotlight. Setting aside the usual denials, suppressions, and cover-ups, there is evidence, mostly from European studies, that cell phone radiation may be a predisposing factor in various brain and eye diseases, so let's assume that is the case. The obvious precautions of using a speakerphone or other hands-free systems seem prudent, but many folks will not implement these measures. The next best thing is to try to implement some sort of shield for the brain and eye to minimize energy absorption, followed by a warning system to the user whenever certain predetermined parameters have been exceeded, increasing the risk of harm. There are all sorts of devices on the market claiming to channel, divert, filter, and otherwise render the RF (Radio Frequency) energy harmless, and many are by far hoaxes. Out of frustration and concern, I collaborated with some friends, one of whom is an RF genius, to come up with some workable solutions. See the side box entitled "CellFrame" for more information.

CellFrame™

The objective was to design some inexpensive ways to reduce the absorption of RF energy by the ear, brain, and eyes, using shielding, attenuation, and reflection methods. An additional goal was to conceive of a warning system for the user, particularly in view of the adaptive power levels that can be generated by modern cell phones. The way that works is if communications with the cell tower are weak, the phone can increase its transmission power level automatically and significantly without the knowledge of the user. Since radiation damage is clearly dose dependent, it would seem prudent to alert the user to this event so that protective action could be taken. From a few brainstorming sessions, a number of designs were generated, several of which make use of the ubiquitous eyeglass frame, hence the trademark CellFrame. A patent application covering the designs has been filed.

For those who live near cell phone towers or other sources of high frequency magnetic fields, an option is to shield yourself from the RF energy. One way to do that is to use electrically conductive paint to paint the room or rooms most used. Once painted, a simple connection between the painted surface and ground will form an RF shield for the entire room. Conductive paints are available that contain copper or carbon particles, and they can be over-painted with suitable sealers and finishes. The website *www.lessemf.com* [237] has information on such paints and methods of making ground connections.

This completes the discussion of physical detoxification protocols, so now let's move on to emotional detoxification.

Chapter 7 - Emotional Detoxification

You may well ask: what is emotional detoxification? The reason this section is here began with some observations by Dr. Klinghardt several years ago while performing heavy metal physical detoxification protocols on patients that were not responding well. In other words, the usual protocols were not producing any significant toxin excretion in clearly toxic patients. However, when these same patients participated in certain types of emotional therapy techniques and released some deep-rooted emotional issues, lo and behold, the toxic metals began to pour out of their bodies. So, what can be described as a mind-body connection was established where emotional detoxification lead to enhanced physical detoxification, an important finding indeed. Since my wife is a licensed psychotherapist, there was quite a bit of interest generated in our household concerning this phenomenon. So began a journey of exploration, and here are my findings. In each instance, I gravitated toward protocols that have demonstrated that they can produce results very quickly.

Family Constellations

I want to begin this discussion with a confession. With my science and law backgrounds, I seem to have a built-in skepticism for any protocol for which I cannot find any plausible explanation. In other words, I do not gravitate towards *woo-woo* stuff. This first protocol, Family Constellations, initially fell into that category and I approached it with a great deal of skepticism. However, after participating in the process, personally benefiting from it, and seeing many others who benefited, I can confidently suggest trying it.

While there are many books on the subject, three in particular present cogent explanations of the work and provide examples. The books are *The Healing of Individuals, Families and Nations* by John L. Payne; *The Language of the Soul* by John L. Payne; and *The Healing Power of the Past* by Bertold Ulsamer. John Payne is a facilitator of Family Constellations in South Africa [239], and Bertold Ulsamer is a facilitator in Germany [240]. The Family Constellation concept was developed by Bert Hellinger, a highly controversial German therapist [241], and it is now being practiced worldwide.

Briefly, when an individual wishes to work on a relationship issue, a theme in their life, or an illness, this technique seeks to look at entanglements within a family system that may be at the root of disruptive life patterns. The protocol is event-oriented inasmuch as personality descriptions or any particular bias or "story" that a client may have is not given much attention. In setting up a constellation, the interest is in *who* is a member of the family system and *what* specifically happened. Events of significance that often have impact on a family system include the early death of parents or grandparents; miscarriages, stillbirths and abortions; murders, tragic and accidental deaths; sudden loss of partner/spouse; adoptions; broken engagements and divorce; war experiences; incest; victims and perpetrators of crime and injustice; family secrets; and individuals who have been forced out of a family or disowned.

During a brief pre-constellation interview, the client is asked about who is in the family and if there have been any specific events that have occurred in the family, such as those listed above. Once the information is gathered, the client is then asked to select participants (usually complete strangers) in the workshop to represent members of their family and any other significant individuals, be they grandparents, uncles, aunts, etc., whose lives may have been impacted by events typical of the list above. Once all of the representatives have been chosen, they are placed intuitively in a standing pattern on the workshop floor space and it is at this point that the constellation comes to life.

The great difference between Family Constellation work and psychodrama or "role play" is that the representatives are not acting out roles according to personality descriptions given by the client. With the set-up of a constellation, the representatives move into and become part of *the knowing field* of the family and remarkably take on the actual feelings and impulses of the real family members. This process is a deep experience not only for the representatives, but also for the client as they watch their family come to life in front of them. Once a Family Constellation is set up, the facilitator first views the set-up in silence, observing both the body language and the pattern that has been created. Very often, the facilitator is able to see indications of certain events that have taken place within the family simply from observing how the representatives are standing in relationship to one another and their overall demeanor, even when the client has made no mention of specific events.

Once these preliminary observations have been made, the facilitator then walks to each representative and asks him or her how he or she is feeling. The feelings reported can be physical descriptions or a wide variety of emotional states. When problems and entanglements are identified, the facilitator then uses healing sentences to bring about resolution. An entanglement is identified when an individual is "tied up" in the fate or business of another. Very often, hidden loyalties are revealed to the extent that a client can be literally carrying and living out both the feelings and the fate of another from their extended family system.

The result of this fascinating process is that what might take years of conventional psychotherapy can sometimes be accomplished in an hour. In the US, the facilitators that I have worked with are JoAnna Chartrand and Dyrian Benz in the Santa Barbara, California area [242]. In other parts of the country, see Bert Hellinger's website for a list of facilitators. Both Drs. Klinghardt and Gruenn, referred to above, have used the Family Workshop protocols as part of their heavy metal detoxification practice, and reported good results. Astute readers may see a subtle connection between the premise of Family Constellations and the premise of Nature's Detox Plan. In the case of The Detox Plan, the objective is alignment between heritage and lifestyle by going back in time to reconcile with our ancestry; in Family Constellations, the objective is alignment between our psyche and our family system by going back in time to reconcile with our ancestry. The analogy is so compelling, and the results so gratifying, that it has rooted this work as an important part of *The Wellness Project.*

Emotional Freedom Technique (EFT)

This simple technique, known as "tapping," can be learned easily at home at no cost, with results in minutes. This is another instance where I don't know why or how it works, but it does. The objective is to resolve quickly at least the symptoms associated with emotional and physical illnesses. It involves a specific sequence of tapping on certain acupuncture points on your head and upper body while you orally repeat a basic formula related to your condition. Developed by Gary Craig, an engineer, this method seems to remove subtle energy blockages in the body and lead to all sorts of emotional and physical healing. At the EFT website [243], you can download instructions, watch a video, and get started tapping away on some of your issues. EFT has been proven successful in thousands of clinical cases, and has been endorsed by many medical doctors and therapists, including Dr. Gruenn, who uses it in his practice. One theory I have as to its efficacy has to do with the analogy of tapping to drumming, discussed further in the lifestyle section, which seems to be the most primitive of human-made external sounds and may be one used by PA as a therapeutic form of healing.

Trauma Healing

Many people traumatized emotionally during episodes of violence or natural disasters often hold on to their experience in a way that takes on a physical life of its own in the form of pain, stiffness, or some distortion in the finely-tuned mechanics of the body. In a real sense, such unresolved traumas add another element of toxicity in the body that needs to be expelled. Peter Levine, a therapist, has developed a theory for dealing with trauma, based on an animal model called the *immobility response*, a survival-enhancing fixed-action pattern that evolved as a protective mode of behavior in prey animals and which is triggered by the perceived imminence of being killed by a predator. As readers know by now, I am a big believer in taking cues from the animal kingdom, and this protocol fits that model. His book *Waking the Tiger* explains the principles and gives examples [244], and his Foundation for Human Experience [245] has a list of practitioners trained in the work.

Section Three - Lifestyle

All the sounds of the earth are like music. - Oscar Hammerstein II

In addition to diet and detoxification, there are many other aspects of PA's lifestyle—to the extent that we know about it or can make educated guesses —that we have abandoned as well. As we grope into our far-distant tropical past for life-style patterns that have relevance to us in today's different world, let's have some fun speculating on what a typical day may have been like for our Paleo Ancestors.

- Awaken by the growing light of dawn.
- Arise from some kind of bedding placed on the ground, maybe outside or in a cave.
- No tooth brushing, mouth washing or flossing, but teeth are naturally perfectly healthy, straight, and free of cavities.
- Begin a day of fruit gathering and animal hunting (while avoiding predators and accidents) barefoot without the use of sunglasses or sunscreen.
- Drinking mineral rich water from streams, ponds, rock and tree depressions, and perhaps taking a dip (no soap).
- The family dress, if any, would probably be limited to primitive loincloths.
- Babies are carried by the mother on gathering trips, and breast-fed on demand, day and night. Pregnant women give birth in a squatting position.
- After eating, individuals squat for bowel movements (no toilet paper needed). If stools are abnormal, remedies are applied to re-establish gut health, including clays and certain anti-parasitic herbs.
- For recreation and relaxation, there would be lovemaking, perhaps primitive drumming and singing, some dancing, and naps.
- After sundown, the clan would retire for at least a nine-hour sleep in a world lit only by moonlight and starlight.

From these general patterns, we can extract ideas that may be useful for us some two million or so years later.

Chapter 8 - Personal Care

By personal care, I mean dental care and substances we put on our skin and hair for various purposes. Let's start with dental care.

Dental Care

The ancients did not use toothpaste and yet, remarkably, from the skeletons that have survived, we find perfect dentition—straight teeth evenly spaced, and no cavities. Along with that, we find wide jaws that accommodate all of the teeth, including wisdom teeth, with no problems. I feel confident that following the Original Diet and Detox protocols will eliminate the tooth decay and gum problems of the modern world, and I do not use any commercial toothpaste, floss or mouthwash.

If we look at animals, such as cats and dogs, we see that they clean their teeth simply by chewing on hides, gristle, and raw bones and some modern indigenous tribes chew on rough bark and twigs as a dental treatment. Taking this as a clue and factoring in the various detox protocols, I arrived at a natural tooth cleaner that is also a detoxifier for the mouth, gums, and the rest of the body – our friend clay.

Ultra-finely-ground clay powder makes a wonderful product for a tooth cleanser, with extremely mild abrasive properties somewhat like baking soda, and no added colorants or sweeteners. Pascalite, the company mentioned earlier as a supplier of an acceptable edible clay, makes such a product called Pasca-Dent which works great [68]. You simply dump some powder in the palm of your hand, wet your toothbrush, stick it in the clay, and use it as toothpaste. There is no significant taste, and besides cleaning your teeth, the clay particles also adsorb bacteria, so after brushing, don't spit it out. Instead, slosh the clay in your mouth for as long as comfortable so it can get between your teeth and around your gums to pick up quantities of oral bacteria. When you are done, you can either spit it out or swallow it.

Mouthwash is also big business, and I have no idea why. It is hardly a solution for bad breath, which is a sign of a gut problem, gum disease, magnesium deficiency, or possibly a sinus or tonsil disorder, all issues that need to be addressed by diet and detoxification. Flossing is a relatively new and somewhat questionable practice. Some dentists feel that flossing can do more harm than good by pushing debris further into gum pockets or hard-to-get areas. I would rather have clay particles between my teeth, on guard 24/7 against a host of nasty stuff. For those who insist on a mouthwash, iodine has been shown to be an excellent choice, particularly for those with root canals or plastic of any kind in their mouth, which fosters fungal overgrowth [246] [247]. Swishing and gargling with a mixture of a few drops of Lugol's solution in mineral water should do the trick. Using the Clayodine concept, I have added a few drops of Lugol's to the clay toothpowder, so I get the effect of an antiseptic toothpaste and mouthwash in one.

Skin Care

We are a society that slathers our skin with tons of toxic stuff in the hope that we can improve its look. My mantra is that, in general, "if it is on the skin, it is also in (the body)." The skin is a great absorber of both good and bad compounds [248]. The threshold question to ask is: why do we need anything on our skin at all? Heavy metal toxins are well known to mess with the skin, causing chronic dryness and all kinds of rashes. An incorrect diet can also cause skin problems like acne and eczema, and fungal overgrowth is well known to cause many skin ailments from athlete's foot to dandruff to ringworm. For clues from MA on skin care, let's peek into the animal kingdom, once again through the lens of Cindy Engel's book *Wild Health.*

Many animals spend a great deal of time tending to their skin, but not for beauty reasons. They are universally plagued by ectoparasites, better known as mosquitoes, gnats, ticks and everything else that bites and stings. In many instances, animals will groom each other, removing pests. In other cases, they have learned how to use natural substances to protect, soothe, and heal the skin. These include covering themselves with certain plant resins and even covering themselves with insects such as ants! In addition, our old friends fruit, dirt, clay, and salt are widely used for skin care, as is sunlight. Some animals will rub fruit over their bodies, including the pulp and rind, which have antiseptic and repellant characteristics. Other animals will roll in mud or cover themselves with clay for soothing effects and to discourage pests. Still other will rub salt on their skin, which kills mites and is beneficial to healing.

Armed with the above, let's see what might work on human skin from Nature. Regarding using fruit on the skin, modernly, alpha hydroxyl acid (AHA), which is fruit acid, is widely used in skin preparations as an exfoliant and remedy for dry skin. A more natural approach might be to cut up some fruit and smear it over the skin on a regular basis. Regarding dirt and mud, I have found that compounds derived from soil and discussed earlier are very soothing to the skin. Morningstar Minerals makes a soil-based product called Derma Boost™ that contains humic acid and is designed to be sprayed on the skin, with good results [52]. Adding spore-forming bacteria to the spray more closely matches the makeup of soil.

Regarding clay, believe it or not, hydrated clay makes a great substitute for soap, eliminating the concern over toxic ingredients. Hydrated clay is clay already mixed with water, and for this application, a pasty consistency works well. You can easily make your own by mixing clay and water to get the desired consistency. Alternatively, the company Nature's Body Beautiful makes a line of clay/water skin cleansers [249], which take some getting used to, as there is no sudsing action. You can put iodine in the mixture as discussed earlier to add antimicrobial action for skin infections. If you insist on soap, the line of baby soaps (and shampoos) from Weleda, a European manufacturer, seems to have a minimum of potentially toxic ingredients [250]. Another choice is soap made with salt, but I am not aware of any made with unrefined ancient dry seabed salt. Those adventuresome readers who are amateur soap makers might wish to make some. In the bacteria detox section, I have already mentioned using an iodine-based hand soap. Finally, as mentioned above, soap nuts can be used as a body soap and shampoo, and instructions are widely available on the internet.

The subject of antiperspirants and deodorants was covered in the discussion of sweating, but for those that insist on using a deodorant, the miracle mineral magnesium is the natural choice. Taking it orally should do the trick, but if not, try wiping the magnesium chloride lotion directly on areas of concern such as the underarms and feet. Bear in mind that magnesium chloride, like ordinary sea salt, causes a burning sensation if put on cuts or irritated skin. An alternative to magnesium chloride lotion is magnesium hydroxide liquid, well known as Milk of Magnesia! Yes, you can swab some unflavored Milk of Magnesia under your arms and it will dry to a powder form and works great as a deodorant .

I cannot find any substantive research on the skin absorption of magnesium hydroxide, so I do not know if it will aid in replenishing body stores through the skin, as does the chloride form. I will tell you, however, that it can be used as a face and body wash with excellent antifungal and antiseptic properties. It is known to relieve dandruff and acne better than most other products. Original Phillips Milk of Magnesia, widely available, can be left on the skin for five minutes or so, and produce positive results for a host of skin problems. This is yet another feather in the cap of magnesium.

Regarding moisturizers, if you are sufficiently detoxified you should not need any since it is the toxins in our body that mess with the natural fatty acids produced by our skin. For those who do need moisturizers, I have come up with an interesting candidate – our friend red palm oil, which you may remember is from an acceptable fruit. The unfortunate problem with this oil is that it stains clothing and temporarily tints the skin slightly orange. However, there is available a palm oil product where the carotenoids that account for the color, and some other unsaturated fatty acids are removed, leaving a colorless paste known as palm oil shortening (not hydrogenated). It works quite well as a colorless moisturizer, and is available from Tropical Traditions [160].

Yet another natural moisturizer that PA would likely have applied to his/her skin is animal fat. Since soap and towels were not available, one can presume that after eating, hands covered in animal fat would have found their way to the hair and skin. More modernly, a product derived from milk fats has been used as a hair and skin moisturizer. It is called ghee, which is made from butter that has been heated, or clarified, and all of the milk proteins are removed, leaving just animal fats. In modern India, where it appears to have originated, ghee is a popular food but is also used topically with great success. I have experimented with it and it is quite soothing to the skin. A popular brand, derived from grass fed cows, is Purity Farms [251]. Although it is a dairy derived product, because all of the potentially offending sugars and proteins such as lactose, whey and casein, have been removed, I see no problem applying it to the skin. Gelatin is related to collagen, a major component of our skin, and taking it is sure to enhance skin tone.

For the most part, cosmetics relate to looking good, reversing the effects of the aging process, and certainly attracting the other sex. Cosmetics are the bottled version of the preening that goes on throughout the animal kingdom—all that peacock strutting and showing off to find a sexual partner to procreate the species. This activity, in one form or another, is obviously built into the genes, humans included. From the study of modern indigenous tribes, we have learned that painting of the body with natural coloring agents is a very old practice, and I recall a particular instance where tribal women used red clay to cover their skin for decorative purposes. This brings me to mineral-based cosmetics.

A recent trend in natural cosmetics is to base them on a variety of naturally colored minerals that have been powdered and combined to match complexions. If you choose to use such a product, you might want some assurance from the manufacturer that no toxic minerals are used, including aluminum and titanium, and that none of the minerals are in nano-particle form, which increases their skin absorption. An example of a manufacturer that provides such products is Earth's Beauty Cosmetics [252].

Sunscreens

In addition to blocking healthy UV light (needed to produce Vitamin D), the other problem with sunscreens is that most of the active ingredients, which are absorbed through the skin, are themselves toxic and can cause DNA damage, which injures skin cells and in fact may contribute to cancer! They have also been found to be hormone disruptors, including interfering with thyroid hormones [253] [254, 255]. This is yet another reason to take iodine supplementation if you are a sunscreen user.

As discussed above in relation to supplementation, the majority of Americans and Western Europeans are way below minimum levels of vitamin D. For more information on this important issue, I suggest reading *The UV Advantage*, by Michael Holick, M.D., of Boston University, who blatantly challenges mainstream thinking in this area regarding the avoidance of UV light exposure. He shows how lack of proper sun exposure can cause serious health problems, such as osteoporosis, colon, ovarian, breast, and prostate cancer, high blood pressure, multiple sclerosis, and depression [92]. I discuss this further in the next section on how to create a healthy living environment.

From my perspective, following the Original Diet and detoxifying will eventually bring you into alignment with your environment, and unless you are an exceptional case where you have moved to a very sunny climate from a heritage country located at a very high or low latitude, your body should be able to handle reasonable amounts of sun without any skin damage. However, if you are very pale- skinned, for example you come from Norway and transplant yourself to Hawaii, you may well have a problem since your naturally low levels of melanin, a trait genetically acquired over generations living in a sun-deprived area, will prevent you from being able to handle a tropical climate without some help.

What should you do in that case or in a situation where you are still detoxing and have not yet reached a healthy equilibrium? Here are my suggestions. First, wear a hat and suitable clothing if you will be getting more than a reasonable amount of UV exposure. Second, be aware of some exciting research using the herb forskolin which, when topically applied, stimulated the formation of additional melanin in rats [256] [257]. This research may produce a new topical treatment to restore melanin in fair-skinned people. Third, be aware of some exciting research into a non-toxic plant- based sunscreen, based on one of my patents (see the box entitled Non-Toxic Plant Based Sunscreen for more information).

Non-Toxic Plant-Based Sunscreen

Some time ago, while I was sitting on the lanai of our Hawaii home, my wife came out and said, “grab your hat, and let’s go for a walk.” At that moment, I looked up at the palm trees and the question popped into my mind: why aren’t these trees wearing a hat. Why can they sit 24/7 in the tropical sun for a hundred years and not burn up? The question took me on a quest into botany and the discovery that we really do not fully understand how plants protect themselves from UV light. An early assumption that it was chlorophyll is incorrect, and the speculation has shifted to some natural compounds of a reddish or bluish color called anthocyanins. These substances are what make blueberries blue and raspberries red, and they are found in high concentrations in our friends - fruit. They are very powerful antioxidants, and are the reason why blueberries have become such a celebrated health food recently. Moreover, the blue and red colors effectively filter UV light. So I decided to create a human sunscreen based on anthocyanins as the active ingredient. My hypothesis was that the colors would filter the light and the antioxidant effect would subdue free radical UV-induced skin damage. If this worked, it would be yet another plus for our use of fruit. After my patent issued (U.S. 6,783,754), I funded the Department of Molecular, Cellular, and Developmental Biology at UC Santa Barbara to undertake skin cell studies to determine the efficacy and dose range for topical anthocyanins used to protect against DNA damage. Preliminary results have been extremely positive, indicating the sunscreen preparation actually stops the DNA damage that could lead to skin cancer. Results of the study are slated for publication in 2009, and grant proposals have already been submitted and funded. Eventually, I hope to interest potential licensees in commercial development.

Fourth, if you insist on using a sunscreen already on the market while waiting for the advanced products, the only one I can suggest is based on zinc oxide as the active ingredient, and it is called UV Natural [258].

Chapter 9 - Living Environment

This section will cover some health issues and possible solutions for the unnatural activity of daily living inside a building, be it a house, apartment or office where you spend a significant part of your time. PA did not have these issues, so we are going to have to come up with some innovative solutions to try to align this environment with our heritage, which is to spend a great deal of our time outside. Let's start with the air we breathe.

Ideally, the objective is to simulate indoors the fresh air of a clean outdoor environment. In today's world, this becomes quite a chore because of the many airborne contaminants inside and outside of our living space. My approach to this is to have a continuously circulating supply of indoor air that has been conditioned to remove toxins, similar to the approach used for water filtration. In my house, I have a rather complete conditioning system sold under the Amana® brand, manufactured by Goodman Manufacturing Co. [259]. The system begins with a forced air gas heater and an outside compressor-based air-cooling system. The entire ductwork was vacuumed to ensure a clean starting environment. Filtration begins with a pleated pre-filter such as the Filtrete® brand Ultra Allergen filter to remove particles around 1 micron in size, and it is on a three-month replacement schedule. This is followed by a whole-house HEPA (High Efficiency Particulate Air) filter using dual carbon cartridges rated to remove particles down to 0.3 microns, including lint, dust, mites, pollen, mold spores, fungi, bacteria, viruses, pet dander, smoke, and grease.

Next in line is a whole-house electronic air cleaner using electrostatic charge to remove these same types of particles down to 0.01 microns in size. Also placed throughout the system are UV air purifiers designed to destroy bacteria, viruses, mold, and volatile organic compounds (VOCs) that either have slipped through the other filters or have collected in the system. The system circulating air fan is kept running continuously, day and night, so the air is continuously filtered. If this sounds like overkill, it is a reflection of the importance I assign to clean air. After all, our interface with the environment is dominated by air, water, and food, so it seems foolish not to pay equal attention to all three.

For those whose indoor environment is not conducive to whole house filtration, room-sized units would be appropriate. I would look for those with a combination of HEPA, electrostatic, and UV filters, and a fan large enough to circulate the room air several times per day. Ceiling fans are also a good idea to keep the air circulating, and in very humid environments, a dehumidifier can aid in reducing mold formation. Air ozonation, which can be used to control mold, is a controversial subject, because large concentrations of ozone can be quite toxic to humans and pets. If mold is a serious and continuous problem, my suggestion is to use ozonators, but only when the area is unoccupied, and then turn them off during occupancy. In our Hawaii home, when we were off-island, we had an ozone generator running continuously along with ceiling fans for circulation, and mold was never a problem.

While it is fine to establish an air filter system, it is equally important to take measures to reduce the amount of contaminants either brought into the home or resulting from the construction of the home itself. Regarding home construction, there are many books regarding the use of home construction materials that have low VOC (Volatile Organic Compound) levels. In addition, I avoid the use of wall-to-wall carpeting, as it usually is manufactured with toxins such as brominated fire retardants (PBDEs) as discussed in the halogen section above, and also acts to accumulate additional toxins by trapping and holding contaminants brought into the home. In my house, I used wood, tile and stone floors partially covered with thin area rugs that are easy to remove and clean. As far as bringing in contaminants, the Japanese custom of removing shoes at the door is a very good one. In addition, for anyone who has been in a toxic environment, such as public parks, golf courses, medical and dental offices, hospitals, factories, etc., it would be prudent to have a place to change clothing and shoes before entering the home. Grass shades are becoming popular for window covering instead of heavy drapes that also tend to accumulate toxins. Of, course, whenever possible, it is a wise idea to open windows to let in sunlight and fresh air, assuming it is not polluted.

I realize that there is a Catch-22 in several of the proposals mentioned above, which increase electricity consumption, raising the issue of increased environmental air pollution from coal- and gas-fired generating stations. Fortunately, fan motors of the type used in air handling systems are now quite efficient and do not consume anywhere near the power used for indoor lighting, our next topic.

Indoor lighting is also filled with a plethora of Catch-22 choices, as we shall see. The ideal objective is to recreate indoors full-spectrum sunlight ranging from infrared to ultraviolet. The classic incandescent bulb produces a yellowish light, is wasteful of energy, and may contain lead in the base. Next, we have the halogen lamp, filled at high pressure with a halogen gas. Remember our halogen detox problem? Well, here it is again. From what little information I can gather of the lighting industry, the gas originally used was our friend iodine, but now they have switched over to *bromine*, one of the dreaded toxic halogens. Halogen lamps are slightly more energy-efficient that plain filament lamps and they are capable of creating light covering most of the visible spectrum. Fortunately, they are produced with thick quartz walls, so that breakage, and possible bromine contamination, is extremely rare. However, their commercial proliferation does contribute to the continued production of bromine, which is already in excess in our environment.

Next, we have fluorescents, which have been around for many years in long-tube form for commercial lighting applications, and are more energy efficient than filament bulbs. More recently, we have compact fluorescent lights (CFLs) that will shortly be mandated for use in new homes, and incandescents will be phased out. Well, in each CFL sits about 5 mg of *mercury*, the most toxic substance of all those discussed in this book. Complicate this with the fact that CFLs are made with a very thin and fragile glass enclosure that is easily broken, spilling mercury. If that happens in your home, you may have a serious problem on your hands. If you do an online search, you will find several horror stories of homeowners who broke these bulbs and were faced with enormous cleanup costs, or ended up contaminating portions of their home. New guidelines are being considered for a warning on the bulbs regarding cleanup procedures.

So here is the environmental Catch-22 for CFLs. Whether or not shifting from incandescent lighting to more energy-efficient fluorescent light will result in a net reduction of mercury emissions due to the displacement of coal-fired electricity generation is questionable at this time. More highly polluting production plants using mercury will need to be established to make fluorescent bulbs to replace incandescent bulbs. In addition, the lack of recycling will put this mercury into landfills where it will contaminate them and leach into drinking water sources. Readers already know my feelings regarding mercury, so I have minimized the use of these bulbs in my home. In the mean time, I have installed low-voltage halogens in readiness for the next wave in interior lighting technology – LEDs.

Full-spectrum LED bulbs are already in production, but the price for total home replacement is still prohibitive. These bulbs are quite energy efficient and at first look, seem to be the preferred choice. However, the fabrication of LED chips is not without environmental issues. Having been involved in semiconductor design and fabrication during the time I was designing and manufacturing solid state relays, I am familiar with the toxic waste disposal issues in that industry, which uses such toxins as arsenic, antimony and hydrofluoric acid (a fluoride compound). Since life is full of informed trade-offs, considering all of the above, my lighting choice at the moment is LEDs, and I intend to start replacement of my halogens in the near future, using full-spectrum whenever possible in an effort to duplicate sunlight. Which brings up the issue of UV light.

It turns out that most residential full-spectrum bulbs on the market are not really full spectrum at all. They deliberately block the ultraviolet portion of the spectrum in the mistaken belief that UV is harmful. From all of the previous discussions in this book regarding UV, vitamin D, and skin cancer, you know that my position is to expose one's body to at least modest amounts of sunlight daily, or else take vitamin D supplements. One way to get UV exposure is by use of a UVB sunlamp, recreating the portion of the solar spectrum responsible for generating vitamin D in the skin. I realize some dermatologist readers out there are cringing at the thought, but mild, non-burning exposure, not designed to give you a deep tan, but to replenish vitamin D, is natural and healthy. This subject is discussed by dermatologist Michael Holick in his book *The UV Advantage*, previously mentioned above [92]. In my home, I have mounted a simple fixture, containing a UVB fluorescent bulb (which I treat with great respect!), on the inside roof of my FIR sauna, and use it for a few minutes several times a week. There are many sources for sunlamps, and one should take care not to go beyond the point that causes a slight pinkness of the skin, and to use eye protection because of the concentrated energy radiated by the lamp. A caveat to those who are, or should be, undergoing detox protocols, your skin may not be able to tolerate any substantial UV exposure until toxins are eliminated, your diet is cleaned up, and normal fatty acid synthesis is restored. In such instance, vitamin D3 supplements are the way to proceed. This brings me to a discussion of sunglasses.

PA obviously did not wear shades, so why do we? Actually, other than the marketing hype and making a fashion statement, I cannot find any good reason for wearing them, sort of like sunscreen. Some in the health field believe that excessive UV light can cause eye diseases such as cataracts. If that is the case, I suggest that UV light may be a necessary, but certainly not sufficient cause, since millions of people who do not wear sunglasses do not get eye disease. My guess is that faulty diet and a body loaded with toxins are the real culprits. The downside to wearing sunglasses is that it interferes with a portion of the endocrine system involving the pineal gland, which is light responsive. We do not fully understand the operation of the pineal gland, but from what we do know, you do not want to mess with it. Some animal tests show that it prolongs lifespan, and it is known to produce melatonin and possibly other hormones that affect the entire endocrine system. I was somewhat shocked to find research that points to the accumulation of *fluoride* in high concentrations in the pineal gland [260], yet another reason to consider the halogen-detox protocol. Another reason to avoid wearing sunglasses is that they can become addictive, because the eyes get used to the reduced light and then become at least temporarily oversensitive to normal sunlight. While there are certainly applications where, for safety reasons, glare-reducing polarized sunglasses should be used, it might be a good idea from a health point of view to forgo sunglasses when they are unnecessary.

Because we rarely base our sleep patterns on sunlight, as PA did, there are a few things that can be done to help keep the body synchronized to natural light. In particular, the release of the hormone melatonin by the pineal gland is stimulated by darkness, and melatonin can contribute to normal sleep patterns. Many of us stay awake in a bright environment until bedtime, not giving the gland much time to adjust to darkness and begin melatonin production. Recent studies have shown that it is the blue portion of the visible light spectrum that shuts off melatonin production [261]. Enterprising companies have developed blue-light blocking eyeglasses and light bulbs that can be used indoors for, say, three hours prior to bedtime to acclimate the pineal gland to darkness. The other portions of the light spectrum do not appear to suppress this hormone production. A company called Photonic Developments [262] makes glasses and light bulbs for this purpose.

Imagine a lifestyle habit that increases alertness, boosts creativity, reduces stress, improves perception, stamina, motor skills, and accuracy, helps you make better decisions, keeps you looking younger, reduces the risk of heart attack, elevates your mood, and strengthens memory. The answer is a daily nap. Research studies continue to show physiological benefits from naps, and I try to nod off for 15 to 30 minutes in the early afternoon. Dr. Sara Mednick has researched and written extensively on the subject, and her website provides the details [263].

Exercise and Relaxation

No book on health seems to be complete without a discussion of exercise. I do not believe exercise can restore an unhealthy person to health, but it certainly can improve their fitness. There has been a lot of research on the life-extending effects of exercise at the cellular level, but if your diet is wrong and you are loaded with toxins, it seems to me that exercise will have a hard time correcting these problems.

What we do know from a study of the animal kingdom and indigenous tribes is that physical exertion in the adult is reserved for obtaining food, dealing with predators including other humans, and reproduction. In fact, energy conservation is an important survival strategy because if you are too fatigued to obtain food, you are history. Since we are privileged not to have to hunt, gather, or evade predators, it takes a conscious effort to get moving, because our immediate survival is not on the line. No wonder exercise is a struggle for many. In search of an answer for this dilemma, I invented and patented a device called the Officizer™, which is described in the side box with that title. In addition to using the Officizer (which I have used daily while writing this book), my personal preferences are walking and resistance training, neither to excess. The use of a pedometer to monitor walking progress can be a helpful motivator.

It is well known that above a certain level of exertion, carbohydrate loading becomes important to avoid severe fatigue. Although PA might have been able to accomplish this by pigging-out on fruit, I truly have a hard time imagining such a scenario on a regular basis. So, for me this is another whisper of wisdom from MA not to overexert. In particular, excessive exercise rapidly depletes the body of magnesium, which may persist for months [100].

The Officizer™

When I was working in an office environment, like many others, I had a room full of exercise equipment at home, which I bought and used for a while. Then one day, sitting at my desk at work, I realized that *now* was when I was ready for some exercise. I wondered, why can't I exercise while I do my work? So I came up with a chair-based exerciser product that straps onto any swivel chair. An adjustable, stretchable band is attached to the center chair post, and at the other end is a bar that resembles a footrest with wheels at either end. You put your feet on it and push, which makes it a combination of a leg press and a leg extension. I designed it to be force balanced so I could push on it without swiveling, which allowed me to read or type at my computer and still be working out. Since it is designed specifically for use in an office environment the Officizer represents a new category of fitness equipment that allows you to be pumping away underneath your desk without anybody knowing what you're doing! The four patents that cover the technology include using the computer you are working on at your desk to monitor your exercise progress. A special mouse design monitors your pulse rate via your fingertip, and a small software program is designed to pop up on the screen every so often to let you know your pulse rate and to spur you on toward meeting pre-established goals. Eventually, I hope to get around to either mass-producing the device or licensing others to do so.

The ideal exercises for us would be based on hunter/gatherer physical behavior, including bending, lunging, squatting, pushing, pulling, and twisting. For those who do tend to overexert when exercising and end up pulling muscles, over-stretching, or otherwise doing some physical injury to their body, I suggest a particular form of chiropractic therapy based on the use of a low-force, spring-driven hammer known as an Activator Adjusting Instrument. The website for this type of therapy lists practitioners proficient in this method and explains how it works [264].

The photos taken by Weston Price of women in the various indigenous tribes around the world have impressed me because of their round faces and bodies, hardly the model look of today. A recent study points to the observation that women with relatively small waists and relatively large hips and thighs store higher body levels of omega-3s, and their children enjoy an edge when it comes to brain development [265]. This might account for the observation that "real women do have curves," in keeping with the movie of a similar name. Perhaps sometime in the future Rubenesque figures will become popular again.

I am not sure whether to characterize making love as exercise, as recreation, or both. However, there is a fascinating book on the subject as it pertains to our genetic heritage written by Jared Diamond, entitled *Why is Sex Fun?,* and it is a great read [266].

Another form of relaxation that seems to be universally portrayed as a pastime of native cultures is drumming. I have no idea if PA drummed, but it is easy to imagine people making drumming sounds as a natural part of living around items such as branches and animal bones that can be knocked together to make noise. There is something primal about drumming that, for me, may be related to the sound of a heartbeat as heard in the womb. Others in the healthcare field have found drumming and other forms of percussion to be particularly healing to those with a variety of health-related problems.

One organization in particular, known as The Rhythmic Arts Project (TRAP), has had great success in working with people with disabilities. Employing drums and percussion, the program teaches and enhances basic life skills such as maintaining focus, using memory, taking turns, developing leadership, using numbers, and following instructions. Issues of spatial awareness, fine and gross motor skills, and speech are also addressed [267]. Once you have music available, dancing is the next logical step, and it is a superb form of exercise that also stretches muscles.

Relating exercise to the air we breathe, there is speculation that the atmospheric oxygen content has been decreasing since the Paleo era, and we do know that the carbon dioxide concentration has more than doubled. This fuels further speculation that increasing the availability of oxygen to the body today might be another way in which to align our environment with our heritage. A few methods of doing so have been suggested. One of them is called EWOT (Exercise With Oxygen Therapy), proposed by Dr. William C. Douglass, who has written a book on the subject [268].

Basically, you hook yourself up to a source of oxygen such as an oxygen tank or an oxygen concentrator using conventional tubing and a nasal cannula, and breathe this oxygen, along with room air, while performing light exercise for 15 minutes. It actually feels quite good to do so, and certainly floods the body's tissues with oxygen, which is normally depleted by exercise. Since you generally need a prescription for oxygen, I presume your MD will want to review this protocol. For details on its use and some case studies, consult the Douglass book.

Section Four - The Future

The significant problems we have cannot be solved at the same level of thinking with which we created them. –
Albert Einstein

The purpose of this section is to summarize a few areas of future research in the field of detoxification that I believe will be most beneficial to the health of our population (and humans in general). Research is sorely needed to develop new non-toxic agents that bind strongly to toxins such as heavy metals, pesticides, certain halogens, fungi, etc. and to escort them out of the body without depositing them elsewhere along the way. Perhaps the alkalinity theory is one answer, but controlled experiments should be conducted as part of a research program. Magnesium's role in the field of detoxification should be researched in great depth, just based on the limited studies that have already been conducted. The treatment of autoimmune conditions should be broadened to include the possibility that they stem from toxins in cells, as opposed to a defective immune system.

In the vaccination arena, rules should be made that anyone dispensing vaccinations must have on hand preservative-free single-dose vials for those who ask for them. Also, alternate vaccination schedules should be provided where inoculations are spread out over time to enable a child's defense system to better deal with them. Lastly, methods for parents to opt out of the programs should be made universal.

In the halogen arena, water fluoridation needs to be banned immediately, and I suggest replacing the fluoride in our water supplies with magnesium! I believe this could have a profound effect on reducing the rates of cardiovascular disease, bone fractures, dental caries, viral infections, and psychological disturbances in our population, and may well be the most important and cost-effective public health measure to be implemented in our lifetime. Of course, whole house water softeners should be banned because they remove magnesium and calcium from the drinking water. Substantial funding should be devoted to high-dose iodine research, covering everything from breast, thyroid, and ovarian cancer to ovarian and breast cysts. Iodine should also be investigated as an alternative to prescription antibiotics and antifungals. The use of bromine should be banned in foods such as bread and soda, as well as in clothing and plastics as a flame retardant. This is another area where private funding will be required, as it has a very negative impact on many commercial enterprises.

I realize that several of the protocols disclosed in this book are not easy to implement, due to a variety of factors such as availability of products, space limitations, and a general reluctance to make radical lifestyle modifications. Therefore, I propose the establishment of neighborhood detoxification centers where many of the diet and detox protocols of The Wellness Project would be made available to the public. A patent application has been filed covering this concept.

It is my intention to devote a portion of the profits from the sale of this book and the licensing of my inventions in the health field to research efforts such as those described above, and I hope there are some readers who will share my passion.

Lastly, I would like to propose a new paradigm for the relationship between a prospective patient and an internist or family doctor. I believe that such a relationship should always begin with the following queries by the doctor:

- Provide a one-week diary of everything you put into or on your body, where the entries are made in real time (record the information when you are ingesting or applying the item). Include how food is cooked, what kind of containers are used, and brand names of products. Be sure to include all medications, supplements, cleansers, and cosmetics.
- Provide a one-week diary of everything that comes out of your body, including frequency of urinations and their color and odor; stool frequency and description, using the Bristol test; and sweat odor.
- Describe your environment – whether mostly indoor or outdoor, age and construction of house, use of carpeting, water supply and filtration, air filtration, use of spas and pools, and use of pesticides.
- Provide complete dental records, including the placement of restorations, materials used, and dates of placement. List all root-canalled teeth, and the age of them.

In addition, I believe the prospective patient is entitled to request from the doctor a list of all of the medications the doctor is taking. The objective is to enable the patient to determine if the side-effect profile of any of these medications might impair the doctor's ability to perform.

As a final note, it is my intention to continue my research into Nature's Detox Plan and generate periodic updates to the information in this book. A website is under construction to facilitate communication with readers, and it will appear at *www.naturesdetoxplan.com.*

Appendix A

Publications

- NASA Tech Brief Document ID: 19660000034 Valve Driver Circuits
- NASA Tech Brief – Triple Redundant Spacecraft Attitude Control System
- NASA Tech Report #JPL-TR-32-1011. DIANA – A Digital-Analog Simulation Program
- NASA Tech Report Document ID: 19680052463 Attitude Control of an Electrically Propelled Spacecraft Utilizing the Primary Thrust System
- NASA Tech Report #JPL-TR-32-1104. The Analysis and Configuration of a Control System for a Mars Propulsive Lander
- NASA Tech Report Document ID: 19670060448. Computer Analysis and Simulation of Mars Soft Landing Descent Control System Combining Inertial and Radar Sensing Techniques
- NASA Tech Report Document ID: 19670006377. Propulsive Planetary Landing Capsule Control System
- NASA Tech Report Document ID: 19670005459 Sterilization of Guidance and Control Systems and Components
- The Analysis and Configuration of a Control System for a Mars Propulsive Lander (Computer analysis and simulation of Mars soft landing descent control system combining inertial and radar sensing techniques) Mankovitz, R J, International Federation Of Automatic Control, Symposium On Automatic Control In Space, 2nd, Vienna, Austria; 4-8 Sept. 1967. P. 21.
- MIL-R-28750 Solid State Relay Military Specification
- EIA RS-433 Solid State Relay Standards
- Author of "THE LAW," a monthly column in Electronic Engineering Times discussing intellectual property law.

AFFILIATIONS AND HONORS:	Intellectual Property Section- CA State Bar
	Eta Kappa Nu- Engineering Honor Society
	Who's Who in California – 1983

Patents

(Health related patents are in **bold**):

PAT. #	Title
6,987,842	Electronic television program guide delivery system using telephone network idle time
RE38,600	Apparatus and methods for accessing information relating to radio television programs
6,783,754	**Plant-based non-toxic sunscreen products**
6,760,537	Apparatus and method for television program scheduling
6,701,060	Enhancing operations of video tape cassette players
6,687,906	EPG with advertising inserts
6,606,747	System and method for grazing television channels from an electronic program guide
6,549,719	Television program record scheduling and satellite receiver control using compressed codes
6,487,362	Enhancing operations of video tape cassette recorders
6,477,705	Method and apparatus for transmitting, storing, and processing electronic program guide data for on-screen display
6,441,862	Combination of VCR index and EPG
6,361,397	**Garments which facilitate the drainage of lymphatic fluid from the breast area of the human female**
6,341,195	Apparatus and methods for a television on-screen guide
6,321,381	Apparatus and method for improved parental control of television use
6,253,069	Methods and apparatus for providing information in response to telephonic requests
6,239,794	Method and system for simultaneously displaying a television program and information about the program

RE37,131 Apparatus and methods for music and lyrics broadcasting

6,154,203 System and method for grazing television channels from an electronic program guide

6,147,715 Combination of VCR index and EPG

6,125,231 Method of adding titles to a directory of television programs recorded on a video tape

6,122,011 Apparatus and method for creating or editing a channel map

6,117,050 Exercise apparatus for use with conventional chairs

6,115,057 Apparatus and method for allowing rating level control of the viewing of a program

6,091,884 Enhancing operations of video tape cassette players

6,086,450 Brassieres which facilitate the drainage of lymphatic fluid from the breast area of the human female

6,072,520 System for improved parental control of television use

6,028,599 Database for use in method and apparatus for displaying television programs and related text

6,010,430 Exercise apparatus for use with conventional chairs

5,995,092 Television system and method for subscription of information services

5,987,213 System and method for automatically recording television programs in television systems with tuners external to video recorders

5,949,492 Apparatus and methods for accessing information relating to radio television programs

5,949,471 Apparatus and method for improved parental control of television use

5,921,900 Exercise apparatus for use with conventional chairs

5,915,026 System and method for programming electronic devices from a remote site

5,734,786 Apparatus and methods for deriving a television guide from audio signals

5,703,795 Apparatus and methods for accessing information relating to radio and television programs

5,690,594 Exercise apparatus for use with conventional chairs

5,677,895 Apparatus and methods for setting timepieces

5,640,484 Switch for automatic selection of television signal sources for delivery of television guide data

5,633,918 Information distribution system

5,581,614 Method for encrypting and embedding information in a video program

5,577,108 Information distribution system with self-contained programmable automatic interface unit

5,561,849 Apparatus and method for music and lyrics broadcasting

5,559,550 Apparatus and methods for synchronizing a clock to a network clock

5,552,837 Remote controller for scanning data and controlling a video system

5,543,929 Television for controlling a video cassette recorder to access programs on a video cassette tape

5,541,738 Electronic program guide

5,526,284 Apparatus and methods for music and lyrics broadcasting

5,523,794 Method and apparatus for portable storage and use of data transmitted by television signal

5,515,173 System and method for automatically recording television programs in television systems with tuners external to video recorders

5,512,963 Apparatus and methods for providing combining multiple video sources

5,499,103 Apparatus for an electronic guide with video clips

5,465,240 Apparatus and methods for displaying text in conjunction with recorded audio programs

5,408,686 Apparatus and methods for music and lyrics broadcasting

5,385,733 Topical preparation and method for suppression of skin eruptions caused by herpes simplex virus

5,382,983 Apparatus and method for total parental control of television use

5,215,748 Topical preparation and method for suppression of skin eruptions caused herpes simplex virus

5,161,251 Apparatus and methods for providing text information identifying audio program selections

5,159,191 Apparatus and method for using ambient light to control electronic apparatus

5,134,719 Apparatus and methods for identifying broadcast audio program selections in an FM stereo broadcast system

5,119,507 Receiver apparatus and methods for identifying broadcast audio program selections in a radio broadcast system

5,119,503 Apparatus and methods for broadcasting auxiliary data in an FM stereo broadcast system

3,691,426 Current Limiter Responsive to Current Flow and Temperature Rise

3,648,075 Zero Voltage Switching AC Relay Circuit

Some health related pending patent applications

Food Compositions and Methods

A Method Of Providing An Eating Plan Having A Very Low Concentration Of Natural Toxins

Silver/Plastic Combination that Binds Hazardous Agents and Provides Anti-Microbial Protection

Iodine Containing Compositions

Systems and Methods for Electrically Grounding Humans to Enhance Detoxification

Apparatus and Methods for Reducing Exposure to RF Energy Produced by Portable Transmitters

Soil Based Composition and Method for Removal of Toxins from Mammals

Methods of Providing to the Public Healthy Diet, Detoxification and Lifestyle Protocols in the Form of Neighborhood Centers

Appendix B - Food and Supplement Schedule

TIME	DIET (See *The Original Diet* for details)	DETOX
Awakening & Bedtime	Mineral Water – 10 oz Dolomite – 1 tablet Optional per magnesium test: Magnesium taurate - 1 cap or tab Fulvic/Humic acid – 1 capsule/AM Spore-formers – 1 capsule/AM ProBoost – 1 packet/PM Sublingual P5P – 2 tablets	Magnesium and Zinc on skin Magnesium Crystals - Bath/Footbath (PM) Sauna (once or twice daily) Grounding Whenever Possible SAMe – 200 to 400 mg For Three Days per 2 Weeks (MYSD): DMPS (every 8hrs or DMSA (every 3-4 hrs); ALA (every 3-4 hrs) For Five Other Days Every 2 Weeks (MYSD): Clay – 2 capsules Fulvic/Humic acid – 1 capsule/PM Spore-formers – 1 capsule/PM
Breakfast & Lunch & Dinner	Animal Foods Fruit Salt Hot Water or Fruit Tea – 8 oz Red Palm Oil – 1 tsp (or: vit. E, K, carotenoids/AM) Eggs (optional) Vitamin C – 500 mg Desiccated Liver – 5 tablets/1 tsp Vitamin D3 – per test results (or UV light) Multimineral – 1 capsule	Apple Pectin – 2 + capsules Vitamin A – 4,000 IU/AM PhosChol (PPC) – 1 gelcap Coenzymated B-Complex/AM (all optional with MYSD detox) Zinc per taste test During the eight days of MYSD detox: Potassium/sodium Citrates – for alkaline urine NAC – 500 mg For three weeks every month (halogen detox): Iodine – per test results Salt/C protocol (optional)
Between Breakfast and Lunch & Between Lunch and Dinner	Mineral Water – 16 oz Dolomite 1 tablet Vitamin C 500 mg Optional: HCl Plus – 1 tab Optional per magnesium test: Magnesium taurate – 1 cap or tab	Charcoal as needed to minimize detox symptoms Every three to six months: Parasite Cleanse – Humaworm

Appendix C - Food and Supplement Resources

(see www.naturesdetoxplan.com for a list of website links)

Food or Supplement	Resource	Website
Salt	RealSalt	www.realsalt.com
Vitamin A; Vitamin D;	Bio-Ae-Mulsion; Bio-D-Mulsion; by Biotics Research	www.bioticsresearch.com
Apple Pectin; Potassium citrate	Apple Pectin USP; Potassium Citrate by Twinlab	www.twinlab.com
Water filters	Doulton Water Filters; Wellness Filters	www.doulton.ca www.wellnessfilter.com
Dolomite; Vitamin C	Dolomite 44 grain; Vitamin C 500 mg by Nature's Plus	www.naturesplus.com
Humic/Fulvic Acids	Immune Boost 77 (capsules) and Vitality Boost HA by MorningStar Minerals; Metal Magnet by PhytoPharmica	www.msminerals.com www.phytopharmica.com
Spore-formers	Flora Balance by O'Donnell Formulas; Lactobacillus Sporongenes by Thorne and Pure Encapsulations	www.flora-balance.com www.thorne.com www.purecaps.com
Edible Clay	Pascalite; Terramin; Redmond Clay	www.pascalite.com www.terrapond.com www.redmondclay.com
Multimineral	Citramin II by Thorne Research	www.thorne.com
Vit K complex; Vit E complex	Super K; Gamma E Tocopherol/Tocotrienols; by Life Extension Foundation	www.lef.org
Liver tablets and powder;	Liver; by NOW Foods	www.nowfoods.com
Red Palm Oil	Tropical Traditions Organic	www.tropicaltraditions.com
Gelatin	Beef Gelatin By Great Lakes Gelatin	www.greatlakesgelatin.com
Magnesium taurate	Magnesium Taurate caps by Cardiovascular Research; Magnesium Taurate 400 tabs by Douglas Labs	www.douglaslabs.com
Magnesium Lotion and bath crystals	Dr. Shealy's Biogenics Magnesium Lotion; Magnesium Chloride Crystals	www.selfhealthsystems.com
Zinc Lotion	Zinc Sulphate Lotion by Kirkman Labs	www.kirkmanlabs.com
Sublingual B-6; Sublingual B	Coenzymated B-6, sublingual; Coenzymated B Complex;	www.sourcenaturals.com

Complex; Zinc; SAMe;	OptiZinc; SAMe; By Source Naturals	
Toilet Squatting Stool	HealthStep by Ginacor	www.healthstep.com
FIR Sauna	High Tech Health	www.hightechhealth.com
FIR heating pads	Thermotex	www.thermotex.com
pH Paper	Micro Essential Lab	www.microessentiallab.com
Clay for baths	Microfine Volclay HPM-20 by American Colloid Company. Distributed by Laguna Clay	www.colloid.com www.lagunaclay.com
Charcoal	Activated Charcoal	www.buyactivatedcharcoal.com
Iodine	Iodoral tablets from Vitamin Research; Lugol's Solution from J. Crow	www.vrp.com www.jcrowsmarketplace.com
Heavy Metal hypersensitivity test	Melisa test	www.melisa.org
Hair Mineral Analysis	Doctor's Data; Ordered from Direct Labs	www.directlabs.com
Iodine skin cleansers	Betadine by Purdue Pharma; widely available from drugstores	www.pharma.com
Stool Tests	Comprehensive Stool Analysis by Genova Diagnostics	www.gdx.net
Parasite cleansers	Humaworm	www.humaworm.com
Grounding equipment	Wrist straps, meters, paint, cords; Bedpads	www.lessemf.com www.earthfx.net
Clay cleansers	Nature's Body Beautiful	www.naturesbodybeautiful.com
Mineral Cosmetics	Earth's Beauty	www.earthsbeauty.com
DMPS	Prescription – supplied by compounding pharmacies	www.amalgam.org
Alpha Lipoic Acid	Lipoic Acid – 25 mg capsules by Kirkman Labs	www.kirkmanlabs.com
DMSA	DMSA – 25 mg capsules by Vitamin Research Products	www.vrp.com
Water Bottles	Glass bottles by ebottle.com	www.ebottle.com
ProBoost	ProBoost Immune System Booster	www.proboostmed.com
NAC, Pantethine, Carotenoids	N-A-C; Pantethine 300; CarotenALL by Jarrow Formulas	www.jarrow.com
PPC	PhosChol by Nutrasal or PPC by Source Naturals or Hepatopro by Life Extension Foundation	www.phoschol.com www.sourcenaturals.com www.lef.org
TOPAS Test	TOPAS test by ALT Bioscience	www.altbioscience.com

EXATEST	EXATEST by IntraCellular Diagnostics	www.exatest.com
Iodine Test	Flechas Family Practice or Vitamin Research Products or Hakala Research Laboratory	www.helpmythyroid.com www.vrp.com www.hakalalabs.com
Cavitat Test	Cavitat by Cavitat Medical Technologies	www.cavitat.com
Soap Nuts soap	Maggie's Pure Land Cleanut by AlmaWin	www.maggiespureland.com www.almawin-usa.com
Magnesium hydroxide	Original Phillips Milk of Magnesia by Bayer Drugs	Widely available

Bibliography

1. Mankovitz, R., *The Wellness Project - A Rocket Scientist's Blueprint for Health*. 2008, Santa Barbara: Montecito Wellness LLC. 360 pp.
2. Mankovitz, R., *The Original Diet - The Omnivore's Solution*. 2009, Santa Barbara: Montecito Wellness LLC. 196 pp.
3. Engel, C., *Wild Health: How Animals Keep Themselves Well and What We Can Learn from Them*. 2002: Houghton Mifflin.
4. Hibberd, A.R., M.A. Howard, and A.G. Hunnisett, *Mercury from Dental Amalgam Fillings: Studies on Oral Chelating Agents for Assessing and Reducing Mercury Burdens in Humans*. Journal of Nutritional & Environmental Medicine, 1998. **8**(3): p. 219-231.
5. Seelig, M.S., *Epidemiology of water magnesium; evidence of contributions to health*. The Magnesium Web Site.
6. Durlach, J., M. Bara, and A. Guiet-Bara, *Magnesium level in drinking water: its importance in cardiovascular risk*. Magnesium in Health and Disease, 1989: p. 173-182.
7. www.mgwater.com, *The Magnesium Web Site*
8. www.ntllabs.com, *Water Testing: National Testing Labs*
9. www.naturesplus.com, *.: Nature's Plus*
10. Rodale, J.I. and H.J. Taub, *Magnesium, the Nutrient that Could Change Your Life*. 1968: Pyramid Books.
11. Kok, F.J., et al., *SERUM COPPER AND ZINC AND THE RISK OF DEATH FROM CANCER AND CARDIOVASCULAR DISEASE*. American Journal of Epidemiology, 2002. **128**(2): p. 352-359.
12. www.doulton.ca, *Doulton Water Filters*
13. www.ppnf.org, *Price-Pottenger Nutrition Foundation*
14. www.wellnessfilter.com, *Wellness Filters*
15. Shotyk, W., M. Krachler, and B. Chen, *Contamination of Canadian and European bottled waters with antimony from PET containers*. Journal of Environmental Monitoring, 2006. **8**(2): p. 288-292.
16. Robbins, W.J. and A. Hervey, *Toxicity of Water Stored in Polyethylene Bottles*. Bulletin of the Torrey Botanical Club, 1974. **101**(5): p. 287-291.
17. Le, H.H., et al., *Bisphenol A is released from polycarbonate drinking bottles and mimics the neurotoxic actions of estrogen in*

developing cerebellar neurons. Toxicology Letters, 2008. **176**(2): p. 149-156.

18. www.ebottle.com, *Glass Bottles*
19. O'Donnell, L., J. Virjee, and K. Heaton, *Detection of pseudodiarrhoea by simple clinical assessment of intestinal transit rate.* BMJ, 1990. **300**(6722): p. 439-440.
20. www.healthstep.com, *HealthStep*
21. Singer, S. and S. Grismaijer, *Dressed to Kill: The Link Between Breast Cancer and Bras.* 1995: Avery Pub. Group.
22. www.intimatehealth.net, *Intimate Health - Brassage*
23. Exley, C., *Does antiperspirant use increase the risk of aluminium-related disease, including Alzheimer's disease?* Molecular Medicine Today, 1998. **4**(3): p. 107-109.
24. Wilson, L., *Sauna Therapy for Detoxification and Healing* 2006, Prescott: L.D. Wilson Consultants.
25. Sylver, N., *The Holistic Handbook of Sauna Therapy.* 2003: Center for Frequency Education.
26. Dantzig, P., *The role of mercury in pustulosis palmaris et plantaris.* Journal of Occupational and Environmental Medicine, 2003. **45**(5): p. 468-469.
27. Dantzig, P.I., *A new cutaneous sign of mercury poisoning?* Journal of the American Academy of Dermatology, 2003. **49**(6): p. 1109-1111.
28. Dantzig, P.I., *Persistent Palmar Plaques—Another Possible Cutaneous Sign of Mercury Poisoning.* Cutaneous and Ocular Toxicology, 2005. **23**(2): p. 77-81.
29. Dantzig, P.I., *Age-related macular degeneration and cutaneous signs of mercury toxicity.* Journal of Toxicology: Cutaneous and Ocular Toxicology, 2005. **24**(1): p. 3-9.
30. Dantzig, P.I., *Parkinson's Disease, Macular Degeneration and Cutaneous Signs of Mercury Toxicity.* Journal of Occupational and Environmental Medicine, 2006. **48**(7): p. 656.
31. Boyd, A.S., et al., *Mercury exposure and cutaneous disease.* J Am Acad Dermatol, 2000. **43**(1 Pt 1): p. 81-90.
32. www.hightechhealth.com, *High Tech Health Saunas*
33. www.drlwilson.com, *Dr. Larry Wilson*
34. www.neuraltherapy.com, *Dr. Dietrich Klinghardt, AANT, KMT, American Association of Neuraltherapy*
35. www.drgruenn.com, *Hans Gruenn MD*

36. www.maggiespureland.com, *Maggie's Pure Land Soap Nuts*
37. www.soapnut.com, *Soapnut Powder*
38. www.almawin-usa.com, *AlmaWin Cleanut*
39. www.thermotex.com, *FIR Heating Pads*
40. Christl, I., et al., *Relating ion binding by fulvic and humic acids to chemical composition and molecular size. 2. Metal binding.* Environ. Sci. Technol, 2001. **35**(12): p. 2512-2517.
41. Liu, A. and R.D. Gonzalez, *Adsorption/Desorption in a System Consisting of Humic Acid, Heavy Metals, and Clay Minerals.* Journal of Colloid And Interface Science, 1999. **218**(1): p. 225-232.
42. Mullen, M.D., et al., *Bacterial sorption of heavy metals.* Appl Environ Microbiol, 1989. **55**(12): p. 3143-3149.
43. Beveridge, T.J. and R.G.E. Murray, *Uptake and retention of metals by cell walls of Bacillus subtilis.* J. Bacteriol, 1976. **127**(3): p. 1502-1518.
44. Fowle, D.A. and J.B. Fein, *Experimental measurements of the reversibility of metal–bacteria adsorption reactions.* Chemical Geology, 2000. **168**(1-2): p. 27-36.
45. www.microessentiallab.com, *Mircroessential Lab- pH paper*
46. Proudfoot, A.T., E.P. Krenzelok, and J.A. Vale, *Position Paper on Urine Alkalinization.* Clinical Toxicology, 2005. **42**(1): p. 1-26.
47. Minich, D.M. and J.S. Bland, *ACID-ALKALINE BALANCE: ROLE IN CHRONIC DISEASE AND DETOXIFICATION.* PHYSIOLOGY. **6**(11): p. 12.
48. www.humichealth.info, *HumicHealth.info*
49. Fung-Jou Lu, H.-P.H.H.Y.Y.Y., *Fluorescent humic substances-arsenic complex in well water in areas where blackfoot disease is endemic in Taiwan.* APPLIED ORGANOMETALLIC CHEMISTRY, 1991. **5**(6): p. 507-512.
50. www.humates.com, *Mesa Verde Resources - Humate Supplier*
51. www.hagroup.neu.edu, *NEU Humic Acid Research Group*
52. www.msminerals.com, *Morningstar Minerals*
53. Huynh A Hong , L.H.D., Simon M Cutting *The use of bacterial spore formers as probiotics.* FEMS Microbiol Rev, 2005. **29**(4): p. 813-35.
54. Ricca, E., A.O. Henriques, and S.M. Cutting, *Bacterial spore formers: probiotics and emerging applications.* 2004: Horizon Bioscience Wymondham, UK.

55. De Oliveira, E.J., et al., *Molecular Characterization of Brevibacillus laterosporus and Its Potential Use in Biological Control.* Applied and Environmental Microbiology, 2004. **70**(11): p. 6657-6664.
56. www.thorne.com, *Thorne Research, Inc.*
57. www.purecaps.com, *Pure Encapsulations*
58. Corsello, S., MD, *Bacillus Laterosporus BOD.* 1996, New York: Healing Wisdom.
59. www.flora-balance.com, *Flora Balance: Bacillus Laterosporus*
60. Diamond, J., *Eat Dirt*, in *Discover Magazine.* 1998. p. pp70-76.
61. Diamond, J., *The Worst Mistake in the History of the Human Race.* Discover, 1987. **8**(5): p. 64-66.
62. Dextreit, R., *Our Earth, Our Cure.* 1974: Swan House.
63. A~, P., *Living Clay.* 2006: Perry Productions.
64. Abehsera, M., *The Healing Power Of Clay.* 2001: Citadel.
65. Callahan, G.N., *Eating dirt.* Emerg Infect Dis, 2003. **9**(8): p. 1016-1021.
66. Graham , C., *The Clay Disciples.* 2006.
67. www.eytonsearth.org, *Healing With Clay, Earth and Mud*
68. www.pascalite.com, *Pascalite Clay*
69. www.terrapond.com, *Terramin Clay*
70. www.redmondclay.com, *Redmond Clay*
71. www.colloid.com, *Amercian Colloid Company - Volclay HPM-20*
72. www.lagunaclay.com, *LagunaClay*2007
73. Heintze, U.L.F., et al., *Methylation of mercury from dental amalgam and mercuric chloride by oral streptococci in vitro.* European Journal of Oral Sciences, 1983. **91**(2): p. 150-152.
74. Rowland, I.R., P. Grasso, and M.J. Davies, *The methylation of mercuric chloride by human intestinal bacteria.* Cellular and Molecular Life Sciences (CMLS), 1975. **31**(9): p. 1064-1065.
75. Trevors, J.T., *Mercury methylation by bacteria.* Journal of Basic Microbiology, 1986. **26**(8): p. 499-504.
76. www.humet.hu, *HUMIFULVATE*
77. www.phytopharmica.com, *PhytoPharmica*
78. Noyes, R., *Handbook of Pollution Control Processes.* 1991: Noyes Publications.
79. Shastri, Y. and U. Diwekar, *Optimal Control of Lake pH for Mercury Bioaccumulation Control.* 2006.
80. www.buyactivatedcharcoal.com, *BUY ACTIVATED CHARCOAL*

81. Said, Z.M., et al., *Pyridoxine uptake by colonocytes: A specific and regulated carrier-mediated process.* Am J Physiol Cell Physiol, 2008: p. 00015.2008.

82. Ershoff, B.H., *Protective Effects of Liver in Immature Rats Fed Toxic Doses of Thiouracil.* Journal of Nutrition, 1954. **52**(3): p. 437.

83. Ershoff, B.H., *Increased Survival of Liver-Fed Rats Administered Multiple Sublethal Doses of X-Irradiation.* Journal of Nutrition, 1952. **47**(2): p. 289.

84. www.nowfoods.com, *NOW Foods*

85. Leklem, J.E. and C.B. Hollenbeck, *Acute ingestion of glucose decreases plasma pyridoxal 5'-phosphate and total vitamin B-6 concentration.* Am J Clin Nutr, 1990. **51**(5): p. 832-6.

86. Wei, I.L., Y.H. Huang, and G.S. Wang, *Vitamin B6 deficiency decreases the glucose utilization in cognitive brain structures of rats.* The Journal of Nutritional Biochemistry, 1999. **10**(9): p. 525-531.

87. www.sourcenaturals.com, *Source Naturals*

88. www.tropicaltraditions.com, *Tropical Traditions - Palm Oil*

89. www.palmoilworld.org, *Palm Oil World*

90. www.jarrow.com, *Jarrow Formulas*

91. www.lef.org, *Life Extension Foundation*

92. Holick, M.F. and M. Jenkins, *The UV Advantage.* 2004: Simon & Schuster.

93. www.vitamindcouncil.com, *Vitamin D Council*

94. Binkley, N., et al., *Low Vitamin D Status despite Abundant Sun Exposure.* Journal of Clinical Endocrinology & Metabolism, 2007. **92**(6): p. 2130.

95. Bastuji-Garin, S. and T.L. Diepgen, *Cutaneous malignant melanoma, sun exposure, and sunscreen use: epidemiological evidence.* British Journal of Dermatology, 2002. **146**(s61): p. 24-30.

96. Elwood, J.M., *Melanoma and sun exposure: An overview of published studies.* International Journal of Cancer, 1997. **73**(2): p. 198-203.

97. Seelig, M.S. and A. Rosanoff, *The Magnesium Factor.* 2003: Avery.

98. Dean, C., *The Miracle of Magnesium.* 2003: Ballantine Books.

99. Whang, R., D.D. Whang, and M.P. Ryan, *Refractory potassium repletion. A consequence of magnesium deficiency*. Archives of Internal Medicine, 1992. **152**(1): p. 40-45.

100. Seelig, M.S., *Consequences of magnesium deficiency on the enhancement of stress reactions; preventive and therapeutic implications (a review)*. 1994, Am Coll Nutrition. p. 429-446.

101. Gontijo-Amaral, C., et al., *Oral magnesium supplementation in asthmatic children: a double-blind randomized placebo-controlled trial.* Eur J Clin Nutr, 2006. **61**: p. 54–60.

102. www.magnesiumresearchlab.com, *Magnesium Research Lab*

103. Arnold, A., et al., *Magnesium deficiency in critically ill patients.* Anaesthesia, 1995. **50**(3): p. 203-205.

104. www.exatest.com, *Magnesium Deficiency - IntraCellular Diagnostics' EXAtest for Minerals Electrolytes*

105. www.bodybio.com, *BodyBio Company*

106. Durlach, J., et al., *Taurine and magnesium homeostasis: new data and recent advances.* Magnesium in cellular processes and medicine. Basel: S Karger publ, 1987: p. 219-38.

107. www.douglaslabs.com, *Douglas Labs*

108. www.selfhealthsystems.com, *Self-Health Systems - Magnesium Lotion*

109. Shealy, C.N., *Holy Water, Sacred Oil.* 2000, Fair Grove, MO: Biogenics.

110. Gaby, A.R., *Intravenous nutrient therapy: the "Myers' cocktail."*. Altern Med Rev, 2002. **7**(5): p. 389-403.

111. Guiet-Bara, A., M. Bara, and J. Durlach, *Magnesium: a competitive inhibitor of lead and cadmium. Ultrastructural studies of the human amniotic epithelial cell.* Magnes Res, 1990. **3**(1): p. 31-6.

112. Soldatovic, D., et al., *Compared effects of high oral Mg supplements and of EDTA chelating agent on chronic lead intoxication in rabbits.* Magnes Res, 1997. **10**(2): p. 127-33.

113. Soldatovic, D., V. Matovic, and D. Vujanovic, *Prophylactic effect of high magnesium intake in rabbits exposed to prolonged lead intoxication.* Magnes Res, 1993. **6**(2): p. 145-8.

114. Djukic-Cosic, D., et al., *Effect of supplemental magnesium on the kidney levels of cadmium, zinc, and copper of mice exposed to toxic levels of cadmium.* Biological Trace Element Research, 2006. **114**(1): p. 281-291.

115. Turnlund, J.R., et al., *Vitamin B-6 depletion followed by repletion with animal-or plant-source diets and calcium and magnesium metabolism in young women.* Am J Clin Nutr, 1992. **56**(5): p. 905-10.
116. Holman, P., *Pyridoxine–vitamin B-6.* Journal of the Australasian College of Nutritional and Environmental Medicine (ACNEM), 1995. **14**: p. 5-16.
117. Schauss, A. and C. Costin, *Zinc as a nutrient in the treatment of eating disorders.* Am J Nat Med, 1997. **4**: p. 8-13.
118. www.bioticsresearch.com, *Biotics Research*
119. www.kirkmanlabs.com, *Kirkman Labs*
120. www.optimox.com, *The Optimox Corporation - Iodorol*
121. www.drbrownstein.com, *Dr. David Brownstein, MD*
122. www.helpmythyroid.com, *Flechas Family Practice*2005
123. Abraham, G.E., *The historical background of the iodine project.* The Original Internist, 2005. **12**(2): p. 57-66.
124. Brownstein, D., *Iodine: Why You Need It, why You Can't Live Without it.* 3rd edition ed. 2007: Medical Alternatives Press.
125. www.helpmythyroid.com, *Flechas Family Practice*
126. www.vrp.com, *Vitamin Research Products*
127. www.jcrowsmarketplace.com, *J.Crow's® Marketplace - Lugol's Solution*
128. www.realsalt.com, *RealSalt*
129. Brownstein, D., *Salt Your Way to Health.* 2007: Medical Alternatives Press.
130. Rooney, J.P.K., *The role of thiols, dithiols, nutritional factors and interacting ligands in the toxicology of mercury.* Toxicology, 2007. **234**(3): p. 145-156.
131. www.twinlab.com, *Twinlab Supplements*
132. Baldewicz, T., *Plasma pyridoxine deficiency is related to increased psychological distress in recently bereaved homosexual men.* 1998, Am Psychosomatic Soc. p. 297-308.
133. www.diagnostechs.com, *Diagnostechs, Inc.*
134. Jefferies, W.M.K., *Safe Uses of Cortisol.* 2004: Charles C. Thomas, Publisher Ltd.
135. Rosanoff, A. and M.S. Seelig, *Comparison of Mechanism and Functional Effects of Magnesium and Statin Pharmaceuticals.* Journal of the American College of Nutrition, 2004. **23**(5): p. 501-505.

136. Cutler, A.H., *Amalgam Illness.* 1999: Andrew Hall Cutler.
137. Imura, N., et al., *Chemical Methylation of Inorganic Mercury with Methylcobalaiin, a Vitamin B12 Analog.* Science, 1971. **172**(3989): p. 1248-1249.
138. www.iaomt.org, *IAOMT International Academy of Oral Medicine and Toxicology*
139. www.toxicteeth.org, *Consumers for Dental Choice*
140. www.informedchoice.info, *Glossary of Vaccines*
141. www.melisa.org, *MELISA® Medica Foundation*
142. Woods, J.S., *Altered porphyrin metabolism as a biomarker of mercury exposure and toxicity.* Can J Physiol Pharmacol, 1996. **74**(2): p. 210-215.
143. Geier, D.A., *A Prospective Study of Mercury Toxicity Biomarkers in Autistic Spectrum Disorders.* Journal of Toxicology and Environmental Health, Part A, 2007. **70**(20): p. 1723-1730.
144. www.directlabs.com, *Direct Labs*
145. www.doctorsdata.com, *Doctor's Data Lab*
146. Cutler, A.H., *Hair Test Interpretation: Finding Hidden Toxicities.* 2004: Andrew Hall Cutler.
147. Ibrahim, D., et al., *Heavy Metal Poisoning: Clinical Presentations and Pathophysiology.* Clinics in Laboratory Medicine, 2006. **26**(1): p. 67-97.
148. www.ccrlab.com, *Clifford Reactivity Test*
149. www.hugnet.com, *Huggins Applied Healing*
150. www.amalgam.org, *DAMS Intl. Dental Amalgam Mercury Solutions*
151. Segermann, J., et al., *Effect of alpha-lipoic acid on the peripheral conversion of thyroxine to triiodothyronine and on serum lipid, protein and glucose levels.* Arzneimittelforschung, 1991. **41**(12): p. 1294-8.
152. Khamaisi, M., et al., *Lipoic acid acutely induces hypoglycemia in fasting nondiabetic and diabetic rats.* Metabolism, 1999. **48**(4): p. 504-10.
153. Barnes, B., *Hope for Hypoglycemia.* 1989, Robinson Press, Incorporated.
154. Waters, R.S., et al., *EDTA chelation effects on urinary losses of cadmium, calcium, chromium, cobalt, copper, lead, magnesium, and zinc.* Biological Trace Element Research, 2001. **83**(3): p. 207-221.

155. De Lucca, A., *In Vitro Inhibitory and Fungicidal Properties of Edta for Aspergillus and Fusarium.* Interscience Conference on Antimicrobial Agents & Chemotherapy Proceedings, 2006: p. 27-30.

156. Duhr, E.F., et al., *HgEDTA complex inhibits GTP interactions with the E-site of brain beta-tubulin.* Toxicol Appl Pharmacol, 1993. **122**(2): p. 273-80.

157. Omura, Y., *Radiation Injury and Mercury Deposits in Internal Organs.* Acupuncture and Electro- Therapeutics Res., Int. J., 1995. **Vol.20**: p. pp. 133-148.

158. Chandra, J., et al., *Modification of Surface Properties of Biomaterials Influences the Ability of Candida albicans To Form Biofilms.* Applied and Environmental Microbiology, 2005. **71**(12): p. 8795.

159. Harrison, J.J., et al., *Metal resistance in Candida biofilms.* FEMS Microbiol Ecol, 2006. **55**(3): p. 479-91.

160. Harrison, J.J., et al., *Metal Ions May Suppress or Enhance Cellular Differentiation in Candida albicans and Candida tropicalis Biofilms?†.* Applied and Environmental Microbiology, 2007. **73**(15): p. 4940-4949.

161. Baklayan, A., *Parasites: The Hidden Cause of Many Diseases.* 2005: Dr. Clark Research Association.

162. Klinghardt, D., *Amalgam/mercury detox as a treatment for chronic viral, bacterial, and fungal illnesses.* Annual Meeting of the International and American Academy of Clinical Nutrition.

163. Djeu, J.Y., et al., *Function associated with IL-2 receptor-beta on human neutrophils. Mechanism of activation of antifungal activity against Candida albicans by IL-2.* J Immunol, 1993. **150**(3): p. 960-970.

164. Worth, R.G., et al., *Mercury Inhibition of Neutrophil Activity: Evidence of Aberrant Cellular Signalling and Incoherent Cellular Metabolism.* Scandinavian Journal of Immunology, 2001. **53**(1): p. 49-55.

165. Perlingeiro, R.C. and M.L. Queiroz, *Measurement of the respiratory burst and chemotaxis in polymorphonuclear leukocytes from mercury-exposed workers.* Hum Exp Toxicol, 1995. **14**(3): p. 281-6.

166. Savage, D.C., *Microbial interference between indigenous yeast and lactobacilli in the rodent stomach.* J Bacteriol, 1969. **98**(3): p. 1278-1283.

167. www.autism.asu.edu, *ASU's Autism/Asperger's Research Program*2007

168. Corey, J.P., C.F. Romberger, and G.Y. Shaw, *Fungal diseases of the sinuses.* Otolaryngol Head Neck Surg, 1990. **103**(6): p. 1012-5.

169. Vaughn, V.J. and E.D. Weinberg, *Candida albicans dimorphism and virulence: Role of copper.* Mycopathologia, 1978. **64**(1): p. 39-42.

170. Weissman, Z., et al., *The high copper tolerance of Candida albicans is mediated by a P-type ATPase.* Proceedings of the National Academy of Sciences of the United States of America, 2000. **97**(7): p. 3520.

171. Kujan, P., et al., *Removal of copper ions from dilute solutions by Streptomyces noursei mycelium. Comparison with yeast biomass.* Folia Microbiol (Praha), 2005. **50**(4): p. 309-13.

172. Truss, C.O., *Metabolic abnormalities in patients with chronic candidiasis. The acetaldehyde hypothesis.* Journal of orthomolecular psychiatry, 1984. **13**(2): p. 66-93.

173. Lieber, C.S., *A LCOHOL: Its Metabolism and Interaction With Nutrients.* Annual Review of Nutrition, 2000. **20**: p. 395-430.

174. Agarwal, D.P. and H.K. Seitz, *Alcohol in Health and Disease.* 2001: Marcel Dekker.

175. South, J.A., *Acetaldehyde: a common and potent neurotoxin.* VRP's Nutritional News, July. Internet, 1997.

176. www.phoschol.com, *PhosChol*

177. Xie, Y., et al., *Ethanol-induced gastric mucosal injury and the protection of taurine against the injury in rats.* Sheng Li Xue Bao, 1999. **51**(3): p. 310-4.

178. Guiet-Bara, A. and M. Bara, *Ethanol effect on the ionic transfer through isolated human amnion. II. Cellular targets of the in vitro acute ethanol action and of the antagonism between magnesium, taurine and ethanol.* Cell Mol Biol (Noisy-le-grand), 1993. **39**(7): p. 715-22.

179. Masuda, M., K. Horisaka, and T. Koeda, *Role of taurine in neutrophil function.* Folia Pharmacologica Japonica, 1984. **84**(3): p. 283-292.

180. Stern, F., et al., *Effect of vitamin B6 supplementation on degradation rates of short-lived proteins in human neutrophils.* The Journal of Nutritional Biochemistry, 1999. **10**(8): p. 467-476.

181. Watanabe, A., et al., *Lowering of blood acetaldehyde but not ethanol concentrations by pantethine following alcohol ingestion: different effects in flushing and nonflushing subjects.* Alcohol Clin Exp Res, 1985. **9**(3): p. 272-6.

182. Craig, J.A. and E.E. Snell, *THE COMPARATIVE ACTIVITIES OF PANTETHINE, PANTOTHENIC ACID, AND COENZYME A FOR VARIOUS MICROORGANISMS.* J. Bacteriol, 1951. **61**: p. 238-291.

183. Firestone, B.Y. and S.A. Koser, *GROWTH PROMOTING EFFECT OF SOME BIOTIN ANALOGUES FOR CANDIDA ALBICANS.* Journal of Bacteriology, 1960. **79**(5): p. 674.

184. www.westonaprice.org, *Weston A. Price Foundation*

185. Iimuro, Y., et al., *Glycine prevents alcohol-induced liver injury by decreasing alcohol in the rat stomach.* Gastroenterology, 1996. **110**(5): p. 1536-1542.

186. Yin, M., et al., *Glycine Accelerates Recovery from Alcohol-Induced Liver Injury.* Journal of Pharmacology and Experimental Therapeutics, 1998. **286**(2): p. 1014.

187. Vidotto, V., et al., *Importance of some factors on the dimorphism of Candida albicans.* Mycopathologia, 1988. **104**(3): p. 129-135.

188. www.proboostmed.com, *ProBoost*

189. Mankowski, Z.T., *Influence of cell-free thymus extracts on the course of experimental Candida albicans infection in mice.* Mycopathologia, 1968. **36**(3): p. 247-256.

190. Rajakrishnan, V., P. Viswanathan, and V.P. Menon, *Adaptation of siblings of female rats given ethanol effect of N-acetyl-L-cysteine.* Amino Acids, 1997. **12**(3): p. 323-341.

191. ÖHman, L., et al., *N-acetylcysteine enhances receptor-mediated phagocytosis by human neutrophils.* Collection sécurité, 1992. **36**(3-4): p. 271-277.

192. Urban, T., et al., *Neutrophil function and glutathione-peroxidase (GSH-px) activity in healthy individuals after treatment with N-acetyl-L-cysteine.* Biomedicine & Pharmacotherapy, 1997. **51**(9): p. 388-390.

193. Vasdev, S., et al., *N-acetyl cysteine attenuates ethanol induced hypertension in rats.* Artery, 1995. **21**(6): p. 312-6.

194. Sprince, H., et al., *Protection against Acetaldehyde Toxicity in the rat by l-cysteine, thiamin and l-2-Methylthiazolidine-4-carboxylic acid.* Inflammation Research, 1974. **4**(2): p. 125-130.

195. Blyth, W. and G.E. Stewart, *Systemic candidiasis in mice treated with prednisolone and amphotericin B. 1. Morbidity, mortality and inflammatory reaction.* Mycopathologia, 1978. **66**(1): p. 41-50.

196. DeMaria, A., H. Buckley, and F. von Lichtenberg, *Gastrointestinal candidiasis in rats treated with antibiotics, cortisone, and azathioprine.* Infection and Immunity, 1976. **13**(6): p. 1761.

197. Larsen, B., et al., *Key physiological differences in Candida albicans CDR1 induction by steroid hormones and antifungal drugs.* Yeast, 1911. **2006**: p. 795-802.

198. Truss, C.O., *The Missing Diagnosis.* 1986.

199. Eaton, K.K., et al., *Abnormal Gut Fermentation: Laboratory Studies reveal Deficiency of B vitamins, Zinc, and Magnesium.* Journal of Nutritional & Environmental Medicine, 2004. **14**(2): p. 115-120.

200. Kariuki, E., R. Ngugi, and J. Muthotho, *Povidone iodine therapy for recurrent oral Candidiasis to prevent emerging Antifungal resistant Candida Strains.* Int Conf AIDS, 2000: p. 13.

201. Shoemaker, R.C., *Mold Warriors.* 2005: Gateway Press.

202. Hume, E.D., *Bechamp or Pasteur?* 2006: DLM.

203. Summers, A.O., et al., *Mercury released from dental" silver" fillings provokes an increase in mercury- and antibiotic-resistant bacteria in oral and intestinal floras of primates.* Antimicrobial Agents & Chemotherapy, 1993. **37**(4): p. 825-834.

204. Lorscheider, F.L., et al., *The dental amalgam mercury controversy—inorganic mercury and the CNS; genetic linkage of mercury and antibiotic resistances in intestinal bacteria.* Toxicology, 1995. **97**(1-3): p. 19-22.

205. Ready, D., et al., *The effect of amalgam exposure on mercury-and antibiotic-resistant bacteria.* International Journal of Antimicrobial Agents, 2007. **30**(1): p. 34-39.

206. Wireman, J., et al., *Association of mercury resistance with antibiotic resistance in the gram-negative fecal bacteria of primates.* Appl Environ Microbiol, 1997. **63**(11): p. 4494-4503.
207. Ready, D., et al., *Oral bacteria resistant to mercury and to antibiotics are present in children with no previous exposure to amalgam restorative materials.* FEMS Microbiology Letters, 2003. **223**(1): p. 107-111.
208. Meinig, G., *Root canal cover-up.* 1994: Bion Pub.
209. Kulacz, R. and T.E. Levy, *The Roots of Disease: Connecting Dentistry and Medicine.* 2002: Xlibris Corp.
210. www.altbioscience.com, *ALT BioScience - TOPAS Test*
211. www.cavitat.com, *Cavitat Medical Technologies*
212. www.lymeinducedautism.com, *L.I.A. Foundation*
213. Davis, I.J., H. Richards, and P. Mullany, *Short Communication Isolation of silver-and antibiotic-resistant Enterobacter cloacae from teeth.* Oral Microbiology and Immunology, 2005. **20**(3): p. 191.
214. www.natural-immunogenics.com, *Natural-Immunogenics - Silver*
215. www.pharma.com, *Purdue Pharma - Betadine*
216. Galland, L., M.D., *Dysbiotic Relationships in the Bowel,* in *American College of Advancement in Medicine Conference.* Spring 1992.
217. Mitsuoka, T., *Intestinal flora and aging.* Nutr Rev, 1992. **50**(12): p. 438-46.
218. www.gdx.net, *Genova Diagnostics*
219. Hunter, J.M., *Geophagy in Africa and in the United States: A Culture-Nutrition Hypothesis.* Geographical Review, 1973. **63**(2): p. 170-195.
220. Shanahan, F., *Probiotics: Promise, Problems, and Progress.* Science. **1**(3): p. 6-8.
221. www.humaworm.com, *HUMAWORM*
222. Shoemaker, R.C., *Desperation Medicine.* 2001: Gateway Press.
223. www.lymephotos.com, *lymephotos*
224. Elliott, D.E., *Does the failure to acquire helminthic parasites predispose to Crohn's disease?* The FASEB Journal, 2000. **14**(12): p. 1848-1855.
225. Potera, C., *Chemical Exposures: Cats as Sentinel Species.* Environmental Health Perspectives, 2007. **115**(12): p. A580.

226. Eriksson, P., C. Fischer, and A. Fredriksson, *Polybrominated Diphenyl Ethers, A Group of Brominated Flame Retardants, Can Interact with Polychlorinated Biphenyls in Enhancing Developmental Neurobehavioral Defects.* Toxicological Sciences, 2006. **94**(2): p. 302.
227. Berkenstam, A., et al., *The thyroid hormone mimetic compound KB2115 lowers plasma LDL cholesterol and stimulates bile acid synthesis without cardiac effects in humans.* Proceedings of the National Academy of Sciences, 2008. **105**(2): p. 663-667.
228. www.cwtozone.com, *ClearWater Tech, LLC*
229. Bryson, C., *The Fluoride Deception.* 2004: Seven Stories Press.
230. Fagin, D., *Second Thoughts about Fluoride*, in *Scientific American.* 2008. p. 74-81.
231. www.fluoridealert.org, *Fluoride Action Network*
232. Abraham, G.E. and D. Brownstein, *Evidence that the administration of Vitamin C improves a defective cellular transport mechanism for iodine: A case report.* The Original Internist, 2005. **12**(3): p. 125-130.
233. Specter, M., *Darwin's Surprise*, in *New Yorker.* January 3, 2008. p. 64-73.
234. Pearson, D. and S. Shaw, *Life Extension: A Practical Scientific Approach.* 1982: Warner Books.
235. Mann, J., *Wipe Out Herpes With BHT.* 1983: MegaHealth Society.
236. www.google.com/patents, *Google Patents*
237. www.lessemf.com, *EMF Safety Superstore*
238. www.earthfx.net, *Earth FX Bed Pads*
239. www.familyconstellations.net, *John Payne - Family Constellations International*
240. www.ulsamer.com, *Bertold Ulsamer*
241. www.hellinger.com, *Bert Hellinger*
242. www.essentialsolutions.info, *Family Constellations - Santa Barbara*
243. www.emofree.com, *EFT Emotional Freedom Technique*
244. Levine, P.A., *Waking the Tiger: Healing Trauma.* 1997: North Atlantic Books.
245. www.traumahealing.com, *Trauma Healing*
246. Bhatt, B.M., et al., *Suppression of Mixed Candida Biofilms with an Iodine Oral Rinse.* 2007.

247. Waltimo, T.M., et al., *In vitro susceptibility of Candida albicans to four disinfectants and their combinations.* Int Endod J, 1999. **32**(6): p. 421-9.

248. Janjua, N.R., et al., *Sunscreens in human plasma and urine after repeated whole-body topical application.* J Eur Acad Dermatol Venereol, 2008.

249. www.naturesbodybeautiful.com, *Nature's Body Beautiful - Clay Cosmeceuticals*

250. www.usa.weleda.com, *Weleda North America*

251. www.purityfarms.com, *Purity Farms - Ghee*

252. www.earthsbeauty.com, *Earth's Beauty Mineral Cosmetics*

253. Hanson, K.M., E. Gratton, and C.J. Bardeen, *Sunscreen enhancement of UV-induced reactive oxygen species in the skin.* Free Radical Biology and Medicine, 2006. **41**(8): p. 1205-1212.

254. Schlumpf, M., et al., *In Vitro and in Vivo Estrogenicity of UV Screens.* Environmental Health Perspectives, 2001. **109**(3): p. 239-244.

255. Schmutzler, C., et al., *The Ultraviolet Filter Benzophenone 2 Interferes with the Thyroid Hormone Axis in Rats and Is a Potent in Vitro Inhibitor of Human Recombinant Thyroid Peroxidase.* Endocrinology, 2007. **148**(6): p. 2835.

256. D'Orazio, J.A., et al., *Topical drug rescue strategy and skin protection based on the role of Mc1r in UV-induced tanning.* Nature, 2006. **443**(7109): p. 340-4.

257. Wickelgren, I., *SKIN BIOLOGY: A Healthy Tan?* Science, 2007. **315**(5816): p. 1214.

258. www.uvnaturalusa.com, *UV Natural Sunscreen*

259. www.goodmanmfg.com, *Goodman Manufacturing Co. - Amana*

260. Luke, J., *Fluoride Deposition in the Aged Human Pineal Gland.* Caries Research, 2001. **35**: p. 125-128.

261. Sasseville, A., et al., *Blue blocker glasses impede the capacity of bright light to suppress melatonin production.* Journal of Pineal Research, 2006. **41**(1): p. 73-78.

262. www.lowbluelights.com, *Photonic Developments - Low Blue Lights*

263. www.saramednick.com, *Take a nap!*

264. www.activator.com, *Chiropractic Activator Methods*

265. Lassek, W., Gaulin, SJ., *Waist-hip ratio and cognitive ability: is gluteofemoral fat a privileged store of neurodevelopmental resources?* . Evol Hum Behav., 2008. **Vol. 29**(Issue 1): p. 26-34.
266. Diamond, J., *Why is sex fun?* 1997: Basic Books.
267. www.traponline.com, *The Rhythmic Arts Project*
268. Douglass, W., *Stop Aging or Slow the Process: How Exercise with Oxygen Therapy (EWOT) Can Help*. 2003, Rhino Publishing.

INDEX

R5

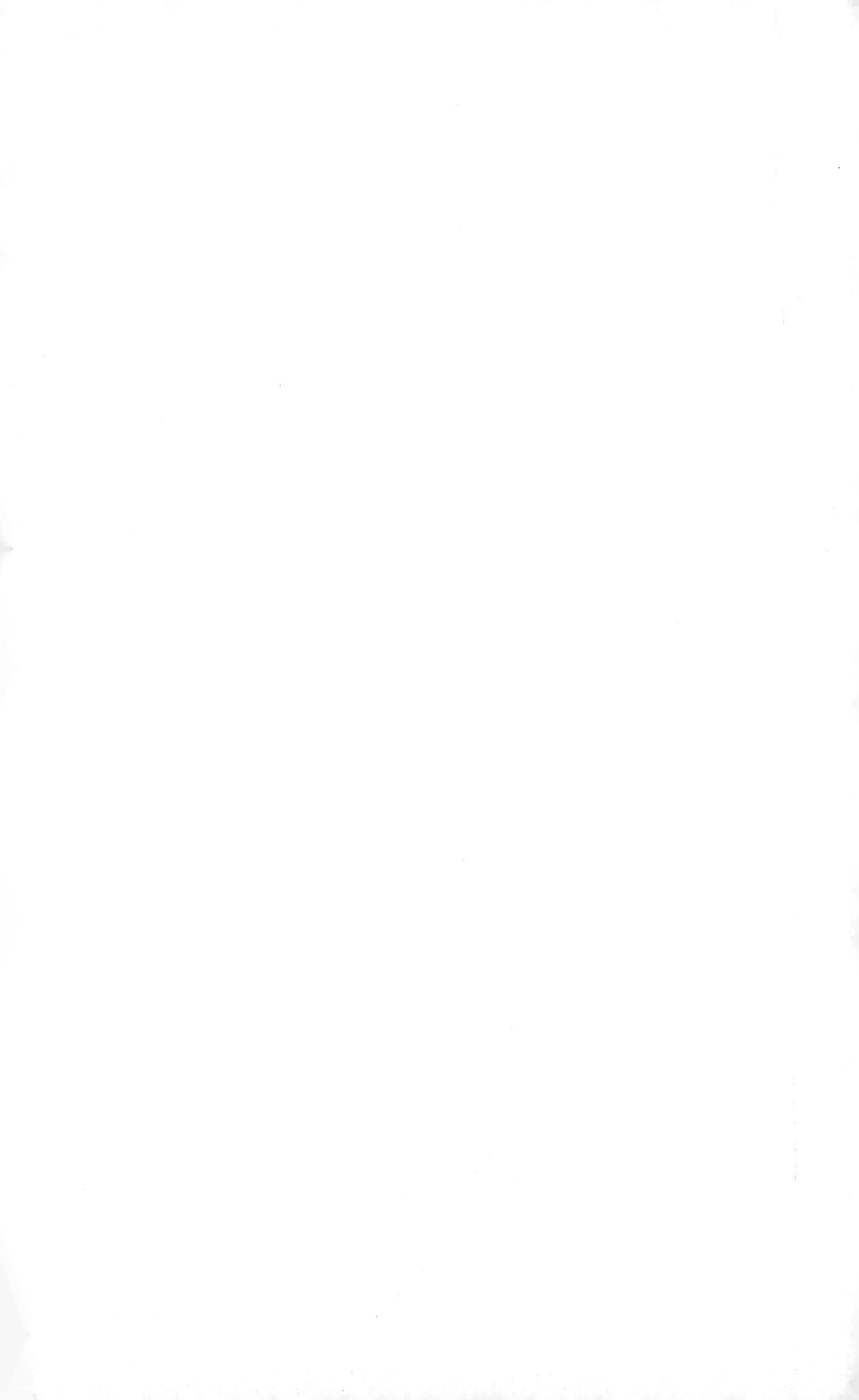

2411043

Made in the USA